PARKINSON'S DISEASE
QUESTIONS AND ANSWERS

FOURTH EDITION

ROBERT A. HAUSER, MD
Professor of Neurology, Pharmacology and Experimental Therapeutics
Director, Parkinson's Disease and Movement Disorders Center
University of South Florida College of Medicine
Chief, Section of Neurology, Tampa General Hospital, Tampa, FL

KELLY E. LYONS, PHD
Research Associate Professor and Director of Research
Parkinson's Disease and Movement Disorder Center
University of Kansas Medical Center
Department of Neurology, Kansas City, KS

RAJESH PAHWA, MD
Associate Professor of Neurology
Director, Parkinson's Disease and Movement Disorder Center
University of Kansas Medical Center
Department of Neurology, Kansas City, KS

THERESA A. ZESIEWICZ, MD
Associate Professor of Neurology
Assistant Director, Parkinson's Disease and Movement Disorders Center
University of South Florida College of Medicine
Tampa General Hospital, Tampa, FL

SPECIAL CONTRIBUTOR
LAWRENCE I. GOLBE, MD
Professor of Neurology,
University of Medicine and Dentistry of New Jersey
Robert Wood Johnson Medical School, New Brunswick, NJ

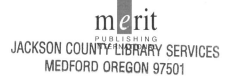

merit
PUBLISHING
INTERNATIONAL

merit
PUBLISHING
INTERNATIONAL

PARKINSON'S DISEASE

QUESTIONS AND ANSWERS

FOURTH EDITION

MERIT PUBLISHING INTERNATIONAL

European address:
35 Winchester Street
Basingstoke
Hampshire RG21 7EE
England

Tel: (+44 0) 1256 841008
Fax: (+44 0)1256 841008
E-mail: merituk@aol.com

North American address:
5840 Corporate Way,
Suite 200,
West Palm Beach,
FL 33407, U.S.A.

Tel: (+1) 561 697 1116
Fax: (+1) 561 477 4961
E-mail: meritpi@aol.com

Web: www.meritpublishing.com

ISBN: 1 873413 68 8

ROBERT A. HAUSER

KELLY E. LYONS

RAJESH PAHWA

THERESA A. ZESIEWICZ

LAWRENCE I. GOLBE

merit
PUBLISHING
INTERNATIONAL

CONTENTS

PARKINSON'S DISEASE

PARKINSON'S DISEASE

QUESTIONS AND ANSWERS

FOURTH EDITION

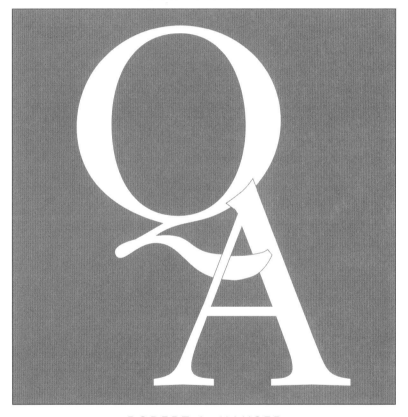

ROBERT A. HAUSER

KELLY E. LYONS

RAJESH PAHWA

THERESA A. ZESIEWICZ

LAWRENCE I. GOLBE

merit
PUBLISHING
INTERNATIONAL

PARKINSON'S DISEASE

CHAPTER 1

INTRODUCTION TO PARKINSON'S DISEASE

Parkinson's disease is a progressive, neurologic disorder caused by a degeneration of dopamine neurons. James Parkinson first described the disease in 1817[1]. Since then, tremendous advances have been made in understanding its pathophysiology and in developing effective treatments. The landmark discovery that levodopa ameliorates symptoms came in the late 1960s. Even today, Parkinson's disease remains one of the few neurodegenerative diseases whose symptoms can be improved with medication therapy. Exciting research into emerging medical and surgical treatments continues at a breathtaking pace. New clues as to its cause are now emerging. This chapter introduces Parkinson's disease, its history, and current concepts of pathophysiology.

What causes the symptoms of Parkinson's disease?

Movement in the human body is produced by the motor cortex. The main motor pathway consists of the pyramidal system, which extends from the motor cortex to the spinal cord. Lower motor neurons carry signals from the spinal cord to muscles to produce movement. The pyramidal system is modulated by the "extrapyramidal" circuit, which includes the substantia nigra, striatum, subthalamic nucleus, the external and internal segments of the globus pallidus, and the thalamus. The extrapyramidal system can either promote or inhibit movement depending on tonic dopamine innervation of the striatum. Normal movement is dependent on appropriate dopamine production by substantia nigra neurons innervating the striatum (figure 1-1).

Parkinson's disease is associated with a massive degeneration of dopaminergic nigrostriatal neurons. When approximately sixty to eighty percent of the dopamine-producing neurons of the substantia nigra are lost, the extrapyramidal system is no longer able to effectively promote movement, and the symptoms of Parkinson's disease appear.

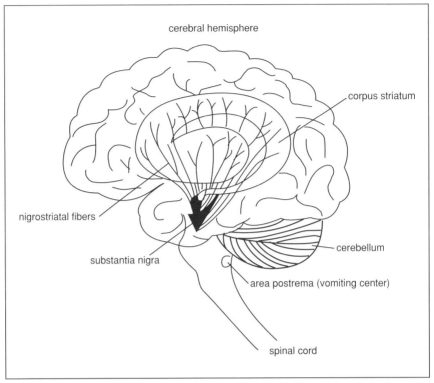

Figure 1-1. *Lateral view of the brain demonstrates dopamine neurons of the substantia nigra innervating the striatum.*

What are the clinical features of Parkinson's disease?

Four main features clinically characterize Parkinson's disease:
1. resting tremor (shaking back and forth when the limb is relaxed)
2. bradykinesia (slowness of movement)
3. rigidity (stiffness, or resistance of the limb to passive movement when the limb is relaxed)
4. postural instability (poor balance).

Onset of symptoms is asymmetric with one limb, usually an arm, affected first. Signs and symptoms then spread to the other limb on that side and later affect the limbs of the opposite side. Resting tremor, bradykinesia, and rigidity are relatively early signs often apparent in the first affected extremity. Postural instability is a late symptom typically emerging ten or more years into the disease.

Other common signs include shuffling gait, stooped posture, difficulty with fine coordinated movements, and micrographia (small handwriting). Secondary features include autonomic dysfunction (constipation, sweating), cognitive decline (dementia), affective disturbances (depression), and sensory complaints including pain in muscles. These will be discussed in greater detail below.

In one recent study, patients reported tremor to be the most troublesome aspect of PD during the first decade following diagnosis. Imbalance was the chief complaint of patients 12-14 years after diagnosis [2].

How did Parkinson's disease get its name?

James Parkinson, a 19th century English physician, was the first to publish an accurate description of the disease in a pamphlet entitled, "An Essay on the Shaking Palsy" [1]. He had encountered several patients who exhibited resting tremor, stooped posture, shuffling gait, and retropulsion (falling backward). He recognized that symptoms progressively worsened, ultimately leading to death from complications due to immobility. The tremor was present with the limbs at rest. He dubbed the disease "paralysis agitans"; paralysis referring to the paucity of movement and agitans referring to the tremor.

Although Parkinson did not identify abnormalities in muscle tone or cognition in his patients, the bulk of his description of the disease was remarkably accurate. The French physician Jean Marie Charcot added muscular rigidity, micrographia, sensory changes, and several other features to Parkinson's original description, and named it after the physician who first clearly described it [3].

Who gets Parkinson's disease?

Parkinson's disease commonly occurs in older individuals, although it may also occur in young adults. It is present worldwide and in all populations [4]. Men have a slightly higher prevalence rate than women [5]. No race or specific region of the world has been found to be completely devoid of the disease.

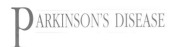

PARKINSON'S DISEASE

What is the mean age of onset of Parkinson's disease?

The mean age of onset of Parkinson's disease is approximately 60 years. It usually occurs in patients over 50 years of age, and onset before age 25 is uncommon. The incidence and prevalence of the disease generally increase with increasing age[5]. Age-specific death rates for Parkinson's disease increased in the elderly in the United States from 1962 through 1984, and decreased in younger age groups[6]. The decreased mortality in younger individuals is likely the result of the introduction of dopamine replacement medical therapy.

How common is Parkinson's disease?

"Prevalence" and "incidence" are two terms used to describe the frequency of a disease. Prevalence refers to the total number of people with the disease in a population at a given time. Incidence is the number of new cases of the disease diagnosed in a population during a given time period. The prevalence of PD increases with increasing age of the population studied. Average crude prevalence rates for Parkinson's disease have been estimated at 120-180 per 100,000 in Caucasian populations[4] and the prevalence of the disease in individuals over 65 years of age is roughly 1%. By the eighth decade, the prevalence of PD in North America and Europe is estimated to be 2-3%[7].

Studies conducted over the last century in Rochester, Minnesota have not uncovered a change in the prevalence of Parkinson's disease in the last fifty years[8]. Incidence rates have been estimated at 20 per 100,000. The lifetime risk of developing PD may be as high as 1 in 40[9].

Does Parkinson's disease occur more frequently in certain locations?

The highest prevalence of Parkinson's disease is in North America and Europe, while the lowest prevalence rates have been found in China, Nigeria, and Sardinia[4]. The Parsi community of Bombay, India was recently found to have a high prevalence rate[10]. The Parsis migrated to India between the seventh and tenth centuries from Iran. They have a closed community, and rarely allow intermarriages with other races or religious groups.

An even higher prevalence rate was reported in Argentina and Sicily[11]. Age-adjusted prevalence rates in Sicily and Junin, a Buenos Aires province in Argentina, was approximately 206/100,000[11,12]. Whether genetic factors in a closed community or some environmental toxin present in the area is causing this high prevalence is unknown.

Is Parkinson's disease more common in Caucasians or African-Americans?

Studies conducted in the United States have generally found a lower prevalence of Parkinson's disease among African-Americans[13]. Even in Africa, the prevalence has been found to be lower in blacks than in whites or Indians[14]. However, in a door-to-door survey conducted in Copiah County, Mississippi, prevalence among blacks was similar to that among whites when relatively loose diagnostic criteria were employed[15]. When more rigid diagnostic criteria were used, whites continued to have a higher prevalence.

Mayeux et al. estimated the prevalence and incidence of PD over a four-year period in a culturally diverse community in New York City, and found a prevalence rate of 107 per 100,000 and an incidence rate of 13 per 100,000 person-years. Age-adjusted prevalence rates were lower for blacks than for whites and Hispanics. However, the age-adjusted incidence rate was highest for black men (black men over age 75 had the highest incidence rate among all groups). A higher mortality rate or delay in diagnosis among black men may account for these findings[16].

Further studies are needed to substantiate the belief that Parkinson's disease is more common in Caucasians and to determine whether access to healthcare or other factors differentially affect the incidence and prevalence of PD in various populations.

What factors are associated with the development of Parkinson's disease?

There is interest in whether exposure to a toxin or multiple toxins might cause Parkinson's disease. It may not be coincidence that James Parkinson's original description of the disease in 1817 occurred at the beginning of the industrial revolution in the United States[17]. Several associations between environmental exposures and Parkinson's disease have been identified including rural living, well-water intake, vegetable farming, exposure to wood pulp, and exposure to pesticides[4].

Some of these associations are controversial and no environmental toxin has been identified that might be causative for most patients with Parkinson's disease. Nonetheless, interest in environmental toxins was greatly bolstered by the discovery that MPTP, a heroin derivative, caused a Parkinson's disease-like illness in young adults who injected themselves with this contaminant[18]. Animals made parkinsonian through injection of MPTP provide a valuable research tool.

What is the prognosis of Parkinson's disease?

Parkinson's disease is a chronic, degenerative disease that usually progresses fairly slowly. Although an average rate of progression can be defined, it is not possible to accurately predict prognosis for an individual patient. Most patients initially do very well on medication for four to six years. Between five and ten years most patients experience medication-related difficulty and many develop poor balance by ten to twelve years. It takes an average of two and a half years to progress from stage to stage (see chapter 4), although this is only a rough guideline[19].

Before the introduction of levodopa, Parkinson's disease dramatically reduced life expectancy. The mortality rate for Parkinson's disease patients was almost three times that of the general population. Treatment with dopamine replacement therapy essentially normalized life expectancy and death rates for Parkinson's disease and non-Parkinson's individuals are now approximately equal[19]. A study conducted in Olmsted County, Minnesota found that patients diagnosed with PD before age 60 had a comparable relative survival rate to the general population, while patients diagnosed at an older age had a lower relative survival rate than expected[20].

What is the basic anatomy and pharmacology of Parkinson's disease?

The major symptoms of Parkinson's disease are due to abnormalities in the extrapyramidal motor circuit. The basal ganglia are subcortical nuclei comprised of three components: the caudate nucleus, the putamen and the globus pallidus (figure 1-2). The caudate nucleus consists of a "head" which lies next to the lateral ventricle, the "body" which lies lateral to the thalamus, and the "tail" which enters the temporal lobe. The putamen and globus pallidus lie between the internal and external capsules, with the putamen situated laterally. The globus pallidus is composed of medial and lateral segments.

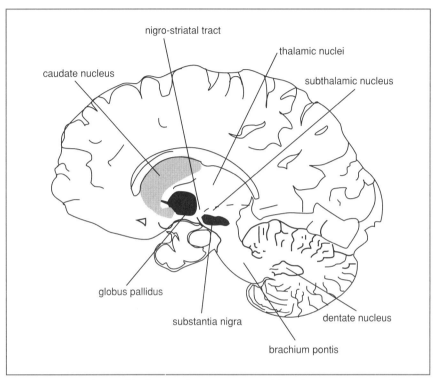

Figure 1-2. *Lateral view of the brain indicating positions of the substantia nigra, caudate, subthalamic nucleus and thalamus.*

Also involved in the extrapyramidal circuit is the substantia nigra. This structure is located in the midbrain, ventral to the tegmentum. It is composed of a pigment-rich area called the "zona compacta" and a relatively cell-poor region called the "zona reticulata". Neurons in the zona compacta are responsible for the production of dopamine, while the zona reticulata primarily produces GABA (gamma-amino-butyric acid).

The ability to produce movement is dependent on a complex motor circuit involving the substantia nigra, basal ganglia, subthalamic nucleus, thalamus, and the cerebral cortex (figure 1-3). Signals from the cerebral cortex are processed through the motor circuit and returned to the same areas by a feedback pathway [21]. The output from the motor circuit is

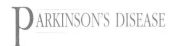

directed through the internal segment of the globus pallidus (GPi) and the substantia nigra pars reticulata (SNr). This inhibitory output is directed to the thalamocortical pathway and suppresses movement.

There are two pathways within the extrapyramidal system: a direct and an indirect pathway. In the direct pathway, outflow from the striatum (putamen and caudate) inhibits the GPi and SNr. The indirect pathway contains inhibitory connections between 1) the striatum and the external segment of the globus pallidus (GPe), and 2) the globus pallidus externa (GPe) and the subthalamic nucleus (STN). The subthalamic nucleus has an excitatory influence on the GPi and SNr. The GPi/SNr sends inhibitory efferents to the ventral lateral (VL) nucleus of the thalamus. Putamenal neurons containing D1 receptors comprise the direct pathway and project to the GPi. Putamenal neurons containing D2 receptors are part of the indirect pathway and project to the GPe. Dopamine activates the direct pathway, and inhibits the indirect pathway.

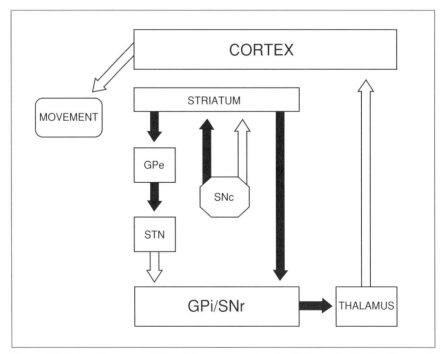

Figure 1-3. *Schematic representation of the normal motor circuit demonstrating the direct and indirect pathways. See text for details. Black arrows represent inhibition and white arrows represent stimulation. SNc = substantia nigra pars compacta; GPe = globus pallidus externa; STN = subthalamic nucleus; GPi = globus pallidus interna; SNr = substantia nigra pars reticulata.*

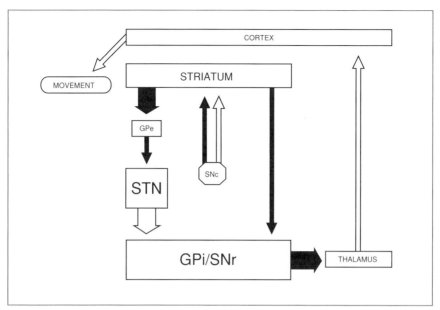

Figure 1-4. *Schematic representation of the motor circuit in Parkinson's disease. Decreased dopamine production by the SNc leads to overinhibition of the thalamocortical pathway. See text for details.*

In Parkinson's disease, decreased production of dopamine by the SNc leads to increased inhibitory output from the GPi/SNr (figure 1-4). This increased inhibition of the thalamocortical pathway suppresses movement. Via the direct pathway, low dopamine levels decrease inhibition of the GPi/SNr, causing overinhibition of the thalamus. Via the indirect pathway, low dopamine levels increase inhibition of the GPe, resulting in "disinhibition" of the STN. Increased STN output promotes GPi/SNr inhibition of the thalamus.

What histopathologic features are associated with Parkinson's disease?

Parkinson's disease involves a degeneration of cells in the substantia nigra pars compacta. The lightly melanized ventral layer in the pars compacta is primarily affected [22]. Clinical manifestations occur when roughly 60% of neurons in this region are lost. Motor symptomatology generally reflects advancing neuronal loss in the substantia nigra [22-25]. In contrast to PD where the greatest loss of neurons is in the ventral layer, with aging there is a greater loss of neurons in the dorsal tier.

It is estimated that with advancing age, 2.1% of neurons in the ventral tier are lost per decade, while 6.9% of neurons degenerate in the dorsal tier[20]. Cell loss in PD is not confined solely to the substantia nigra but also affects the locus ceruleus, thalamus, cerebral cortex, and autonomic nervous system. Neurotransmitter abnormalities involve the cathecholaminergic and serotonergic systems as well as the dopaminergic system.

The pathological determination of Parkinson's disease includes the identification of Lewy bodies[22]. These are eosinophilic, concentric, hyaline inclusions present in the cytoplasm of some remaining substantia nigra pars compacta neurons. They can also be found in the locus ceruleus, autonomic neurons, and other areas. Lewy bodies consist of a dense center and a pale staining, peripheral halo. The outer layer consists of cytoskeletal elements.

It was recently discovered that alpha-synuclein is a major structural component of Lewy bodies[26]. This is an important observation because abnormalities in the gene for alpha-synuclein cause PD in some families (see chapter 4). Lewy bodies have also been found in other degenerative disorders and in some elderly individuals without parkinsonian features. The presence of Lewy bodies at autopsy in some "normal" individuals may suggest that they had preclinical Parkinson's disease, and would have developed signs and symptoms if they had lived longer. Incidental Lewy bodies are present in about 1% of the non-parkinsonian population dying at 50-59 years of age[27,28]. The prevalence of incidental Lewy bodies rises to 10% for individuals dying at 80-89 years of age. This compares with a 1-2% prevalence of PD in the 80-89 year old age group, suggesting that Lewy bodies are present during a preclinical period before symptoms become apparent[27,28]. Neurodegenerative diseases marked by Lewy bodies include corticobasal degeneration, motor neuron disease, ataxia telangiectasia, subacute sclerosing panencephalitis, and Hallevorden Spatz disease[27].

What is the neurochemistry of Parkinson's disease?

Dopamine and other cathecholamines are synthesized from tyrosine by the following pathway:

tyrosine --> 3,4-dihydroxyphenylalanine (DOPA) --> dopamine --> norepinephrine --> epinephrine.

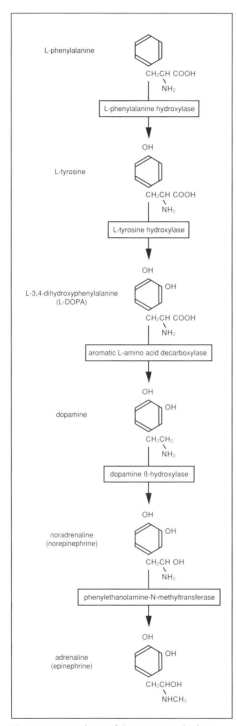

Figure 1-5. *Synthesis of dopamine and other catecholamines.*

The rate-limiting step in the formation of dopamine is the hydroxylation of tyrosine to form DOPA. This step is catalyzed by the protein tyrosine hydroxylase (figure 1-5).

Tyrosine hydroxylase is a marker of dopamine neurons. It is decreased in the substantia nigra of Parkinson's disease patients. Dopamine and its metabolites, homovanillic acid (HVA) and dihydroxyphenylacetic acid (DOPAC), are reduced in the striatum, the primary target of dopamine neurons[29]. Dopamine loss is more extensive in the putamen than in the caudate[30]. Dopamine levels are also reduced in the hypothalamus, mesolimbic, and mesocortical areas.

Once formed, two enzymes metabolize dopamine: monoamine oxidase (MAO), which deaminates dopamine intraneuronally, and catechol-O-methyl transferase (COMT), which methylates dopamine outside the neuron[31] (figure 1-6). MAO exists in two forms: MAO-A and MAO-B. MAO-B is the predominant form in the brain and is found on the outer membrane of mitochondria. MAO-B inhibitors increase levels of striatal dopamine. COMT methylates dopamine extraneuronally by catalyzing the

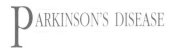

transfer of a methyl group from S-adenosyl-L-methionine to the m-hydroxy group of dopamine. Dopamine is also deactivated by neuronal reuptake via the dopamine transporter.

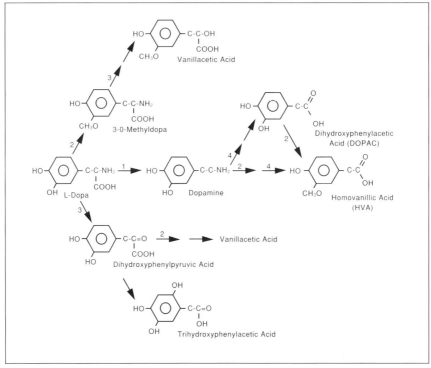

Figure 1-6. *Metabolism of levodopa and dopamine. 1=aromatic amino acid decarboxylase; 2=catechol-O-methyltransferase; 3=tyrosine aminotransferase; 4=monoamine oxidase.*

What are the different types of dopamine receptors?

Receptors are macromolecules composed of proteins located on neuronal membranes (figure 1-7). The two main types of dopamine receptors are D1 and D2 [32,33]. Dopamine functions by modulating the direct and indirect pathways of the extrapyramidal motor circuit through its effect on D1 and D2 receptors. Dopamine receptors are linked to a guanine nucleotide-binding protein (G-protein), to form a complex, which interacts with adenyl cyclase to control formation of the second messenger, adenylate cyclase (figure 1-8). The D1 receptor family includes D1 and D5 receptors, while D2 includes D2, D3, and D4 receptors (figure 1-9). Receptors in the D1 family increase cyclic AMP, while those in the D2 family reduce cyclic AMP [32,34]. D2 receptor activation is important in the anti-parkinsonian response to dopamine agonist medications. The role of D1 receptor activation in the response to medications is less clear.

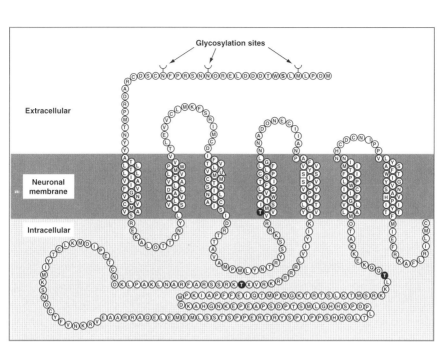

Figure 1-7. *Structure of D2 receptor. Each circle represents an amino acid. Black circles represent phosphorylation sites.*

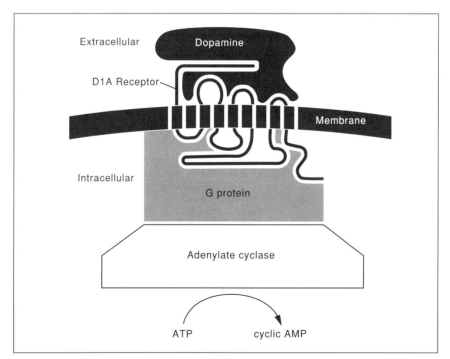

Figure 1-8. *D1 receptor. The receptor is linked to a G protein to control the synthesis of the second messsenger, cyclic AMP.*

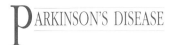

	D1	D2			
	A	B	A	B	C
Currently used term					
Previously used term	D1	D5	D2	D3	D4
Location (high concentrations)	Striatum Nucleus accumbens Amygdala Olfactory bulb	Hippocampus Hypothalamus	Striatum Nucleus accumbens Substantia nigra Olfactory bulb	Hypothalamus Nucleus accumbens Olfactory bulb	Frontal cortex Midbrain Medulla
Action (information is limited to biochemical indexes)	Increases cyclic AMP	Increases cyclic AMP	Reduces cyclic AMP Opens potassium channels Closes calcium channels	Reduces cyclic AMP	Reduces cyclic AMP

Figure 1-9. *Distribution and function of dopamine receptors.*

Are there tests available to diagnose Parkinson's disease?

The diagnosis of Parkinson's disease is made by clinical evaluation and there are currently no simple, widely available laboratory tests that make the diagnosis. Fluorodopa positron emission tomography (PET) is a useful index of striatal dopaminergic function [35] but is expensive (usually not covered by insurance) and not widely available. Single photon emission computerized tomography (SPECT) using radioisotopes that bind to the dopamine transporter on nigrostriatal neuron terminals is also emerging as a useful modality [36]. Further development of SPECT technology may provide a widely available and relatively inexpensive diagnostic tool in the near future.

CHAPTER 2

ETIOLOGY OF PARKINSON'S DISEASE

LAWRENCE I. GOLBE
Special Contributor

Although the cause of Parkinson's disease is unknown, the modern consensus is that most cases of PD are the product of a combination of genetic and environmental factors. Under this "multifactorial" hypothesis, PD is the result of several factors in a given individual. The precise combination of causes varies from one individual to the next. This could explain how a disorder with a prominent genetic component occurs in sporadic fashion in a majority of cases. Similarly, the multifactorial hypothesis could explain how a disorder with a major exogenous toxic component displays no clear geographical or occupational predilection.

To what extent is Parkinson's disease an inherited disorder?

Only about 20% of individuals with PD know of an affected first-degree relative. For controls without PD, the figure is about 5%[1]. The ratio of these figures, a measure of familial aggregation, is lower than that of well-recognized adult-onset genetic disorders such as Huntington's disease. However, convincing evidence for an important but subtle genetic component in some or perhaps all cases of PD has emerged in the last decade.

A powerful measure of the genetic influence on disease is to compare the concordance rates in monozygotic (MZ)(identical) twins to that of dizygotic (DZ)(non-identical) twins. A large, early study reported a 4.7% concordance rate in 43 MZ twin pairs and a 5.3% concordance rate in 19 DZ twin pairs[2]. A subsequent re-examination of those data using more inclusive diagnostic criteria[3] found that the concordance rate for MZ twins rose to 12% while the concordance rate for DZ twins remained unchanged at 5.3%. This ratio suggested a strong genetic factor with low penetrance.

A larger study using a database of U.S. World War II veterans found a similarly low concordance rate in MZ and DZ pairs (MZ 16%, DZ 11%, risk ratio=1.4)[4]. However, in 16 pairs of twins with diagnosis at or before age 50 years, all 4 MZ pairs, but only 2 of 12 DZ pairs, were concordant (MZ 39%,

DZ 11%; RR=3.6). These findings suggest little or no genetic component when the disease begins after 50 years of age, but genetic factors appear to be very important when the disease begins at or before age 50.

This study, despite its thoroughness, used only clinical examinations to determine if an individual had PD. Positron emission tomography (PET) using labeled fluorodopa ([18F]-DOPA) is more sensitive for PD in that it can detect preclinical dopamine neuron loss.

The most thorough PET study evaluated unaffected co-twins in pairs where only one had clinical signs of PD (clinically discordant) at baseline and again an average of 4 years later[5]. At baseline, a significantly higher concordance rate for decreased striatal dopamine function was found in the 18 monozygotic clinically unaffected co-twins compared to the 16 dizygotic unaffected co-twins (55% versus 18%). This constituted unprecedented evidence for a major genetic component to PD. Even more convincing was the second [18F]-DOPA PET scan in the same subjects, which showed a clear decline in dopaminergic function over time in all of the asymptomatic monozygotic co-twins. The clinically unaffected dizygotic co-twins declined no faster than controls.

The issue of genetic contribution to apparently sporadic PD was examined in a very different way by researchers in Iceland, where centuries of genealogical records document distant familial relationships among most of the living population[6]. They randomly chose a number of patients with sporadic PD and a similar number of controls. They then randomly formed pairs of patients and pairs of controls and examined the genealogical records to quantify the closeness of the relationship within each pair. The relationships proved to be much closer for the patients than for the controls, suggesting that PD, at least in Iceland, tends to be hereditary, but with low penetrance, thereby producing the appearance of sporadic occurrence.

Are there families in whom Parkinson's disease is clearly inherited?

One large family with highly penetrant, autosomal dominant, autopsy proven PD, originated in the town of Contursi in the Salerno province of southern Italy[7]. Its 60 affected individuals were characterized by early age of disease onset (mean age of 47.5 years), rapid progression (death at mean age of 56.1 years), paucity of tremor and a good response to dopamine medication therapy. A few had cortical dementia that is quite unusual for PD, but for the most part, the range of clinical pictures was similar to that of sporadic PD. Linkage analysis incriminated a region in chromosome 4q21-23[8]. Sequencing of several candidate genes in that region revealed an A for G substitution at base 209 of the alpha-synuclein gene[9]. This was considered a candidate only because a fragment of the alpha-synuclein protein was known to occur in amyloid plaques of Alzheimer's disease. The single base-pair missense mutation codes for a substitution of threonine for alanine at amino acid 53 (A53T).

After the discovery of the A53T mutation in the Contursi kindred, workers the world over sought that mutation in patients with sporadic PD or with familial PD where the family was too small for linkage analysis on its own. The A53T mutation was found in 12 small families, all of Greek origin[10]. A German family was found to have a different point mutation in the alpha-synuclein gene (a substitution of C for G at base 88, producing a substitution of proline for alanine at amino acid 30)[11]. The alpha-synuclein mutations causing PD are together termed "PARK1."

What is alpha-synuclein?

Alpha-synuclein is a presynaptic nerve terminal protein found abundantly in the brain, particularly in the olfactory bulb and tract, hypothalamus, and substantia nigra. The details of its function remain unknown, but it is involved in maintenance and intracellular transport of dopaminergic vesicles before they release dopamine into the synapse. PARK1 mutations disrupt the a-helical portion of the alpha-synuclein molecule, substituting a beta sheet configuration. This appears to produce abnormal aggregation of alpha-synuclein[9].

The mechanism by which alpha-synuclein aggregation leads to cell death is not known, but may be related to the ability of an early stage of such aggregates ("protoaggregates" or "oligomers") to create pores in plasma membranes, thereby impairing cellular function[12].

Are abnormalities of alpha-synuclein found in idiopathic Parkinson's disease?

One of the most exciting recent advances is the discovery that alpha-synuclein is a major component of Lewy bodies, a histopathologic hallmark of PD[13]. This suggests that abnormal aggregation of alpha-synuclein occurs in all PD and may be an etiologic factor.

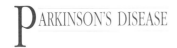

Although sporadic PD (and most familial PD) is not caused by a mutation in the alpha-synuclein gene, there is active investigation into other proteins that interact with alpha-synuclein, including those that guide, promote or prevent aggregation of the protein. There is evidence that dopamine itself promotes alpha-synuclein aggregation [14,15]. This could explain the predilection of the PD disease process for dopamine neurons. Certain commonly used pesticides [16] and metals [17] have a similar effect, perhaps explaining the epidemiologic association of PD with those exposures.

There may be so many causes of abnormal alpha-synuclein aggregation that minimizing the population's exposure to them would be impractical. However, if alpha-synuclein aggregation is a common pathogenetic factor in all PD, treatments might be developed to prevent it directly or to disrupt the pathways by which it causes dopamine cell death. Although investigators are just beginning to unravel these mechanisms, there is a good chance that this discovery represents the breakthrough that will ultimately lead to a cure or prevention for PD.

How have alpha-synuclein animal models helped?

The first useful models of PD involved injection of 6-hydroxydopamine into the striatum of rodents, or the use on non-chemical procedures, to create striatal lesions. These models aided in understanding the neurophysiology of the disorder and testing treatments, but not in mimicking the molecular changes underlying human PD. The MPTP model in rodents and primates described below was more faithful to the neurochemistry of PD and has advanced our understanding significantly.

Even better animal models are emerging from the discovery of the involvement of alpha-synuclein in human PD. Drosophila [18], and to a lesser extent mice [19], in which the normal human alpha-synuclein gene has been "knocked in" have recently provided excellent models of the molecular events involving alpha-synuclein aggregation, Lewy body formation and dopamine neuron cell loss.

Alpha-synuclein models have demonstrated, for example, that heat-shock proteins interfere with alpha-synuclein aggregation and its toxicity [20] and that geldanamycin, an inducer of heat-shock protein, prevents the neuronal degeneration completely [21]. Such insights could easily lead to a prevention for PD.

What is the parkin gene?

Mutations in the parkin gene cause many of the cases of autosomal recessive juvenile parkinsonism (AR-JP)[22-24]. AR-JP is characterized by early onset parkinsonism (before age 40 and often before 30), slow disease progression, improvement following sleep, good response to levodopa therapy and levodopa-induced dyskinesias[22], without dementia or autonomic symptoms. The gene was originally found in Japanese families[22,23] but has since been found in many other populations[25].

The parkin gene is on the long arm of chromosome 6 (6q25.2-q27). The N-terminal of the normal protein resembles ubiquitin, while the C-terminal may function as a zinc-finger protein[26]. Pathologically, AR-JP is marked by neuronal loss in the substantia nigra and locus ceruleus, without Lewy bodies. A huge range of mutations in the large parkin gene has been described, from large deletions to single base substitutions. AR-JP caused by parkin mutations ordinarily requires that both copies of chromosome 6 carry the same mutation (homozygosity) or that each copy carry a different mutation (duplex heterozygosity). But individuals with only one copy of a small parkin mutation (heterozygosity) can have late-life onset of symptoms and receive a diagnosis of idiopathic PD[27].

Parkin protein is a ubiquitin ligase, an enzyme that cuts the polyubiquitin chain as part of the process that delivers defective or worn-out proteins to the proteasome for disposal and recycling of their component amino acids. Parkin dysfunction therefore permits accumulation of an as-yet unidentified waste protein, which presumably aggregates to produce neuronal loss. There is mounting evidence that sporadic PD also involves dysfunction of the ubiquitin-proteasome system[28], possibly via impaired breakdown of alpha-synuclein[29]. Better understanding of this role could soon offer excellent opportunities for pharmacologic intervention in the disease process.

What other genes are associated with PD?

Eight other genes associated with strongly familial PD, PARK3 through PARK10, have been identified with regard to their general chromosomal location. This was accomplished through total genome searches using linkage analysis. Only one has been localized to a specific gene. PARK5 is a mutation in the gene for ubiquitin carboxy terminal ligase 1 (UCHL-1)[30]. However, many geneticists dispute the association of this gene with PD, as only two affected members of one family carried it.

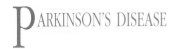

A potentially very interesting PD-causing gene is PARK3. It was mapped to chromosome 2p13 via linkage analysis of the Iowa kindred, a family that immigrated to the US from northern Europe[31]. The specific gene has not yet been identified and PARK3 appears not to be a common cause of PD outside of this kindred. However, a locus identical to PARK3 appears to play a role in determining onset age of PD as determined by analysis of a large cohort of PD-concordant siblings[32]. The eventual cloning of the PARK3 gene and the elucidation of its pathophysiology could prove a major advance in understanding sporadic PD, just as have the identification of PARK1 and PARK2.

Dozens of other genetic variants have been associated with sporadic PD, not via a total genome search, but by comparing the frequencies of alleles of candidate genes between patients and controls. This technique is prone to false positives and each newly announced association must be viewed in this light. For example, the first such association implicated the gene for CYP2D6, an hepatic detoxification enzyme. Despite a few confirmatory studies, the weight of the evidence is now against such an association.

How are other PD genes being sought?

Although the best way to find PD-associated genes is via linkage analysis of large families with multiple cases of PD, that method has the disadvantage of requiring at least 10 affected members who can provide DNA samples, which for a late-life-onset condition is difficult. Furthermore, the cause of a highly penetrant form of PD may have little relevance to the cause of sporadic or weakly familial (i.e., low-penetrance) hereditary PD. The allelic association method mentioned above is one solution, but it has the disadvantages of frequent false positive results and an ability to analyze only the one gene deemed a candidate.

A method that avoids these pitfalls is to gather a large series of co-affected pairs of siblings and to perform a whole-genome search. Approximately 400 pairs are necessary given present technology. At least four such projects are underway and each has incriminated several chromosomal loci so far. These await confirmation and sequencing of candidate genes.

What is the oxidation hypothesis?

The oxidation hypothesis suggests that chemical reactions involving electron transfers may cause or contribute to progression in Parkinson's disease. Oxidation reactions normally take place in the body and play important roles in

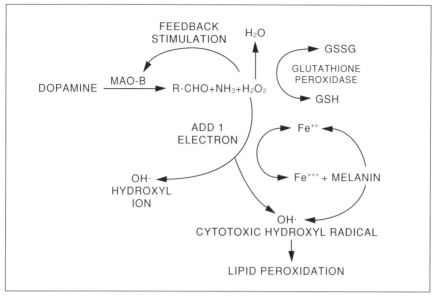

Figure 2-1. *Formation of cytotoxic hydroxyl radical. Dopamine's oxidative metabolism leads to the formation of hydrogen peroxide (H_2O_2). Hydrogen peroxide is normally cleared by glutathione. If protective mechanisms are overwhelmed, hydrogen peroxide can accept an electron to form hydroxyl ion (OH-) and cytotoxic hydroxyl radical (OH•). Melanin and iron may serve as electron donors and create site-specific oxidative stress.*

the production of high-energy compounds. A molecule is "oxidized" when it donates an electron, and "reduced" when it receives an electron. Oxidation reactions may lead to the formation of free radicals, highly reactive and unstable molecules that contain an unpaired electron.

Dopamine's oxidative metabolism leads to the formation of hydrogen peroxide. Hydrogen peroxide is normally rapidly cleared by protective mechanisms including glutathione. If protective mechanisms are overwhelmed, hydrogen peroxide can be reduced to form the highly reactive hydroxyl free radical, which can react with membrane lipids in the brain, leading to lipid peroxidation and cell damage. The brain may be particularly vulnerable to oxidative damage due to its large oxygen consumption, abundant material for lipid peroxidation, and limited ability to regenerate[33]. An oxidating environment promotes the aggregation of alpha-synuclein[34, 35], providing another possible route to neuronal degeneration.

Are protective enzymes decreased in Parkinson's disease?

Parkinson's disease patients have decreased levels of reduced glutathione in the substantia nigra, without an increase in oxidized glutathione[36]. These

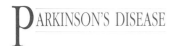

findings are thought to be specific to Parkinson's disease, and are not observed in conditions such as multiple system atrophy. It is unclear whether decreased glutathione levels are caused by abnormalities in its synthesis or metabolism and the exact localization of the deficiency is also unknown. Decreased levels of reduced glutathione may compromise protective mechanisms, allowing hydrogen peroxide to become available to form hydroxyl radicals.

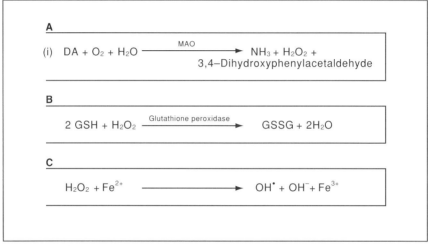

Figure 2-2. *A) Metabolism of dopamine by MAO. B) Clearance of H_2O_2 by reduced glutathione (GSH), thereby preventing the interaction of H_2O_2 with iron. C) The Fenton reaction. H_2O_2 that has not been cleared can accept an electron from Fe2+ to form the highly reactive hydroxyl radical (OH•).*

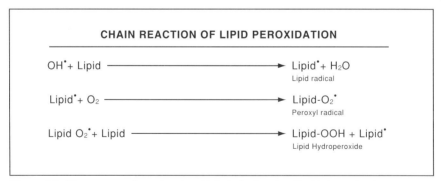

Figure 2-3. *The sequence of reactions in which the hydroxyl radical initiates lipid peroxidation.*

What is the role of neuromelanin and iron in Parkinson's disease?

Oxidation reactions are facilitated by transition metals including iron, copper, and manganese. The brain contains a higher concentration of iron than any other metal, and it is probably essential for normal brain function. Iron accumulates in the normal brain until about age 20, after which time levels remain fairly constant. Iron is normally bound to the protein transferrin, which acts as a buffer to limit electron transfers. Parkinson's disease patients have increased iron levels in the substantia nigra pars compacta and decreased levels of transferrin, thus making iron more available for participation in oxidation reactions[37]. Neuromelanin in the substantia nigra has a high affinity for iron, and may serve as an electron source, thereby promoting the formation of free radicals[38]. The presence of neuromelanin may confer site-specific vulnerability on substantia nigra neurons. Iron also promotes the aggregation of alpha-synuclein, providing another explanation for the iron-PD association[17].

Is there evidence of increased lipid peroxidation?

Evidence of increased lipid peroxidation has been found in the substantia nigra of Parkinson's disease patients. There are higher levels of malondialdehyde, an intermediate in lipid peroxidation, and lipid hyperoxides[39].

What is the role of superoxide dismutase in Parkinson's disease?

Superoxide dismutase is a scavenger enzyme, which may protect cells from free radical damage[40]. High levels of superoxide dismutase have been found in the substantia nigra on mitochondrial membranes of normal individuals[41]. Copper-zinc-dependent superoxide dismutase messenger RNA is higher in mesencephalic neurons containing neruomelanin compared to other neurons, suggesting that melanized neurons require a defense against free radicals[42]. Increased superoxide dismutase levels are found in Parkinson's disease patients irrespective of gender, age, or treatment[43]. This may reflect an effort to defend against increased free radical production.

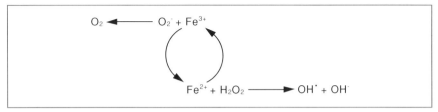

$$O_2 \longleftarrow O_2^{\cdot} + Fe^{3+}$$

$$Fe^{2+} + H_2O_2 \longrightarrow OH^{\cdot} + OH^{-}$$

Figure 2-4. *Redox cycling of iron from its oxidized to its reduced state can drive oxidation reactions, thereby promoting the formation of cytotoxic free radicals.*

What is MPTP?

MPTP, or 1-methyl-4-phenyl-1,2,3,6-tetrahydropyridine, is a chemical that causes a clinical syndrome closely mimicking idiopathic Parkinson's disease. This was first observed in a chemist who was synthesizing illicit substances in his lab. He developed parkinsonism after intravenous injection of a mixture of 1-methyl-4-phenyl-4-hydroxypiperidine or MPPP, a potent meperidine analogue, and MPTP [44]. Autopsy revealed dopamine neuron degeneration specifically within the substantia nigra.

Several other individuals who self-injected MPTP were later identified and examined [45]. Shortly after intravenous injection, these patients developed visual hallucinations, stiffness, limb jerking, and immobility. This stage was also marked by a sense of euphoria. Bradykinesia progressed for up to three weeks after injection. The ensuing chronic stage was marked by all of the motor features of Parkinson's disease, as well as some infrequent findings including eyelid apraxia, freezing, and dystonia. Levodopa administration brought about marked improvement in parkinsonian signs and symptoms. Side-effects of chronic dopamine replacement therapy such as dyskinesia occurred more rapidly than in idiopathic Parkinson's disease [45]. Autopsies revealed selective destruction of the dopamine neurons of the pars compacta of the substantia nigra. MPTP has since been utilized to create an excellent animal model of Parkinson's disease for research.

MPTP is actually a protoxin that is oxidized to the true toxin MPP+ by the enzyme monoamine oxidase type B. MPP+ accumulates in mitochondria, and interferes with the function of Complex I of the respiratory chain. The extrinsic oxidation hypothesis suggests that an environmental protoxin is oxidized to a toxin that causes Parkinson's disease. Searches for such an environmental toxin have not identified a chemical that is likely to cause Parkinson's disease in idiopathic cases. Still, the identification of a chemical causing a syndrome so similar to Parkinson's disease is a landmark discovery that continues to provide new insights into possible etiologic mechanisms.

What is the role of pesticides?

Soon after the identification of MPTP as a dopaminergic toxin, epidemiologists aware of the chemical resemblance of MPTP to some commonly used pesticides looked for occupational or residential risks associated with PD. A pesticide-PD association was found, but it is not clear that this is not merely a proxy for a different causal agent often encountered by the same rural population that tends to encounter pesticides[46]. Still, it is intriguing that rotenone and paraquat, two common pesticides, damage mitochondrial function and each promotes aggregation of alpha-synuclein[17]. Administration of rotenone to rodents produces alpha-synuclein aggregation and neuronal loss in a pattern similar to human PD[17].

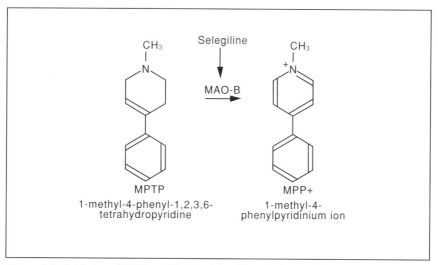

Figure 2-5. *Oxidation of MPTP to MPP+ is inhibited by selegiline, a selective inhibitor of MAO-B.*

Perhaps the best current theory of PD etiology is a subtle, long term exposure to pesticides in individuals with genetically determined deficiencies in detoxification and with marginal mitochondrial reserve, also on a genetic basis.

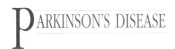
What is the role of mitochondria in the pathogenesis of Parkinson's disease?

The toxic metabolite of MPTP, MPP+, inhibits complex I of the electron transport chain, causing a parkinsonian syndrome in affected individuals and laboratory animals[47]. This raises the question as to whether complex I is abnormal in idiopathic Parkinson's disease. Several laboratories have reported deficiencies of mitochondrial electron transport chain complex I in the substantia nigra of Parkinson's disease patients[48]. A blinded study examining platelet mitochondrial activity in early untreated Parkinson's disease patients and age- and sex-matched controls found lower complex I activity in platelet mitochondria in PD patients[49]. This suggests that chemical defects in Parkinson's disease may be widely expressed in the body and that the mitochondrial defect is genetically determined.

What is the role of smoking in the etiology of Parkinson's disease?

Cigarette smokers have approximately 40% less risk of developing PD relative to non-smokers[50]. The most plausible explanation is that smoking causes an induction of protective enzymes, but this is unproven. A competing hypothesis is that the very early stages of PD entail a deficiency

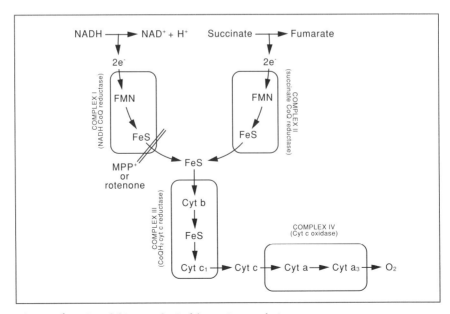

Figure 2-6. *MPP+ inhibits complex I of the respiratory chain.*

in the dopaminergic addiction-reward system. Smoking or nicotine treatment provides no symptomatic benefit to patients with PD and of course, healthy nonsmokers, even those with a family history of PD, should not start smoking for the purpose of preventing PD.

What other environmental exposures may help cause Parkinson's disease?

Some aspect of rural living is associated with PD. Exposure to pesticides or herbicides, well water use and farming experience have all been implicated in various surveys. Which of these, if any, is the actual culprit is unclear. A history of minor head trauma is also more common in PD [46]. Coffee drinking reduces PD risk by about 30%, possibly on the basis of adenosine receptor blockade. [51]

Does aging cause Parkinson's disease?

Many elderly individuals exhibit some degree of bradykinesia and 90% of all cases of PD start after age 40. In fact, the likelihood of developing PD increases with each successive decade of life. Does the mere passage of time allow a disease with a long "incubation period" to manifest itself? Or are PD and aging qualitatively the same thing, one being merely an accelerated form of the other?

Pathologic studies have documented a loss of neurons in the substantia nigra pars compacta with advancing age [52], as well as a decrease in the cross-sectional size of the midbrain [53]. The rate of decline of dopamine neurons in elderly persons has been estimated to be as high as 10% per decade [53,54]. Levels of tyrosine hydroxylase, the rate-limiting enzyme in the synthesis of dopamine, also decrease with advancing age [53].

The evidence against the "aging hypothesis" of PD is stronger. Loss of dopamine neurons in the substantia nigra pars compacta in normal aging is greatest in the medial ventral and dorsal tiers. In Parkinson's disease, neuronal loss in greatest in the lateral ventral tier, followed by the medial ventral and dorsal tiers [55].

Even more convincing, there is important neuronal loss in the caudate and putamen in aging, while those neurons, the sites of the dopamine receptors in the nigrostriatal pathway, remain intact in PD. This could explain the failure of the bradykinesia of aging to respond to dopamine replacement with levodopa[56]. Furthermore, Lewy bodies, the pathologic hallmark of degenerating neurons in PD, do not occur in large numbers in normal aging.

Therefore, although aging may contribute to a loss of dopamine neurons, it does not provide an explanation for the pattern or rate of dopamine neuron loss in idiopathic Parkinson's disease. This does not exclude the possibility that age-related changes may enhance susceptibility to etiologic factors or permit their expression. But this is very different from a conclusion that PD is merely an acceleration of the aging process.

Is there a role for viruses in the etiology of Parkinson's disease?

Suspicion that viruses might play a role in the pathogenesis of Parkinson's disease was prompted by the occurrence of postencephalitic parkinsonism following the outbreak of encephalitis lethargica (von Economo's encephalitis) from 1917-1926. However, there is no clear evidence linking idiopathic Parkinson's disease to a viral infection. Virologic studies performed on brains of Parkinson's disease patients using electron microscopy and immunofluorescent studies have failed to detect viral particles or antibodies[57]. Several studies have demonstrated an increase in herpes simplex antibody levels in patients with Parkinson's disease[58] but a causal relationship seems unlikely. An old theory linking PD with the influenza pandemic of 1918 has also been thoroughly discredited.

CHAPTER 3

DIFFERENTIAL DIAGNOSIS OF PARKINSON'S DISEASE

The differential diagnosis of Parkinson's disease is vast. Causes of secondary Parkinsonism include medications and toxins, cerebrovascular disease, infection, trauma, metabolic abnormalities, and brain neoplasms (figure 3-1). The "atypical parkinsonisms" are a group of degenerative disorders with clinical features that include bradykinesia and rigidity, but differ from Parkinson's disease both pathologically and clinically. The atypical parkinsonisms are characterized clinically by lack of tremor, early speech and balance difficulty, and little or no response to dopamine medication therapy. This group of diseases includes progressive supranuclear palsy, corticobasal degeneration, and the multiple-system atrophies.

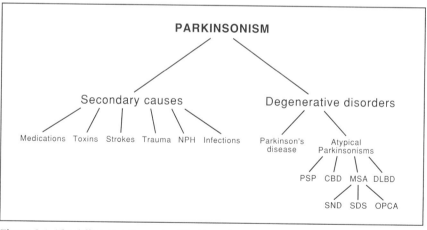

Figure 3-1. *The differential diagnosis of Parkinsonism.*
NPH=Normal Pressure Hydrocephalus
SND=Striatonigral Degeneration
PSP=Progressive Supranuclear Palsy
SDS=Shy-Drager Syndrome
CBD=Corticobasal Degeneration
OPCA=Olivopontocerebellar Atrophy
MSA=Multiple System Atrophy
DLBD=Diffuse Lewy Body Disease

The multiple system atrophies are marked clinically by a combination of extrapyramidal, pyramidal, autonomic and cerebellar abnormalities. Included in the multiple system atrophies are striatonigral degeneration, olivopontocerebellar atrophy, and Shy-Drager syndrome. This chapter will examine the differential diagnosis of Parkinson's disease, including characteristic features used to help recognize various diseases and possible therapies.

When should I be most suspicious that I am dealing with something other than Parkinson's disease?

One should always consider the differential diagnosis of Parkinson's disease before making a diagnosis. In all cases it is important to exclude the possibility of medication-induced parkinsonism. When dealing with young patients one's index of suspicion for other disorders should be especially high as Parkinson's disease is generally a disease of older individuals. In patients with bradykinesia and rigidity, the combination of the absence of tremor and little or no response to dopaminergic medications greatly increases the likelihood that the correct diagnosis is not Parkinson's disease.

Which medications cause parkinsonism?

Many pharmacologic agents can produce features of parkinsonism, including tremor, bradykinesia, rigidity, shuffling gait, and speech disturbances. These include dopamine-blockers such as the neuroleptics and antiemetics, as well as dopamine depletors such as reserpine and tetrabenazine. The gastrointestinal motility drug metochlopramide has both peripheral and central dopamine antagonism, and is probably the most underrecognized cause of medication-induced parkinsonism today.

Other drugs that can cause extrapyramidal signs include lithium[1], alpha-methyl-dopa[2], and some of the tricyclic antidepressants[3]. Antiepileptic medications can induce cerebellar symptoms[4] and valproic acid can cause tremor[5]. Patients presenting with parkinsonism who have recently taken any of these medications should be observed for at least six months off the medication before a diagnosis of Parkinson' s disease is made[6].

Which toxins cause parkinsonism?

Toxins known to cause parkinsonian symptoms include manganese, carbon monoxide, methanol, ethanol, and MPTP or 1-methyl-4-phenyl-1,2,3,6-tetrahydropyridine, a synthetic heroin derivative [7].

Which neurologic conditions mimic Parkinson's disease?

ARTERIOSCLEROTIC PARKINSONISM was first described by Critchley in the 1920's. "Vascular parkinsonism" is usually characterized clinically by bradykinesia and rigidity without tremor, and there may be other neurologic evidence of stroke [8]. Patients with multiple strokes may experience a step-wise progression of symptoms. An MRI should confirm the presence of cerebrovascular disease, although precise MRI criteria for a diagnosis of vascular parkinsonism are lacking. Tremor caused by cerebrovascular disease is uncommon, although there have been reports of unilateral tremor caused by vascular lesions in the thalamus [9]. Dystonia may also be caused by strokes involving the basal ganglia.

INFECTIONS, including viruses such as HIV, and tuberculosis can cause parkinsonian signs. Postencephalitic parkinsonism is an historic example of an infectious cause of parkinsonism. "Encephalitis lethargica" or "von Economo's disease" occurred in an epidemic from 1919-1926. It commonly affected young adults in their 20s and 30s, but also affected a substantial number of children [10]. Early symptoms included fever, mental changes, and neurologic deficits consistent with encephalitis. Mortality rates were high. Those who survived were left with various neurologic deficits in the chronic encephalitic phase. Parkinsonism developed weeks to years after the acute phase [11].

Postencephalitic parkinsonism included bradykinesia and rigidity. Additional characteristic features were oculogyric crises with involuntary upward deviation of both eyes, and sleep rhythm disturbances. The parkinsonian features were often relatively stable and limited in progression. Pathologic changes were seen in the substantia nigra, subthalamic nucleus, and hypothalamus [10]. Very few postencephalitic parkinsonism patients are alive today owing to the more than seventy years that have elapsed since the outbreak of encephalitis lethargica.

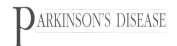

TRAUMA can also cause parkinsonism. Boxers who endure repeated trauma to the head may develop a syndrome of dementia, parkinsonism, pyramidal, and cerebellar signs [12]. "Dementia pugulistica" refers to the cognitive changes boxers experience years after the trauma occurred. Multiple concussions cause diffuse axonal injury secondary to acceleration-deceleration forces affecting the brain. It is postulated that repeated head trauma may initiate dopamine neuron degeneration. Pathologically, there is a loss of pigmented neurons in the substantia nigra, in the absence of Lewy bodies. Neurofibrillary tangles without senile plaques are found in the cerebral cortex [13].

NORMAL PRESSURE HYDROCEPHALUS is an acquired condition leading to changes in mentation, gait disturbances, and urinary incontinence. Patients develop bradykinesia without tremor. Gait apraxia mimics the shuffling gait of Parkinson's disease. The diagnosis is made by a combination of clinical and imaging findings. MRI demonstrates hydrocephalus with the lateral ventricles dilated out of proportion to the cortical sulci and Sylvian fissures. Radionuclide cisternagram may demonstrate slow clearance of CSF. Some, but not all, patients will respond to shunting. Unfortunately, it is not currently possible to predict which patients will respond.

TUMORS and other mass lesions can occasionally cause parkinsonian features. This can be due to direct compression of the nigrostriatal tract by tumor or by stretching due to hydrocephalus.

What neurologic diseases are in the differential diagnosis of Parkinson's disease?

ESSENTIAL TREMOR (familial tremor) is characterized by a postural tremor of the upper extremities not caused by a pharmacologic agent [14]. The disease usually occurs in patients who are over the age of forty and transmission is autosomal dominant with approximately 70% of patients reporting a family history of tremor. The tremor is predominantly postural, often with a kinetic component. The postural component is observed with the arms outstretched and the kinetic component with the arms in motion such as when performing the finger-to-nose test. Tremor frequency is often higher than that of Parkinson's disease, with a range of 4 to 12 Hz [15].

Essential tremor usually involves the upper extremities, is relatively symmetric, and is best seen with the arms outstretched, resulting in a flexion-extension or pronation-supination movement of the hands. The tremor slowly worsens over time[16]. Stressful activities transiently increase the amplitude, and ingestion of alcohol may temporarily reduce it. The arms are usually affected, while the legs and trunk are normally spared. Essential tremor commonly includes a head or voice tremor, whereas tongue, jaw, and lip tremors are more characteristic of Parkinson's disease.

Other clinical manifestations of Parkinson's disease such as bradykinesia and rigidity are not present in essential tremor. Fifty to eighty percent of patients diagnosed with essential tremor will experience a good clinical response to medications such as propranolol or primidone[17]. However, this response is somewhat non-specific as the tremor of Parkinson's disease may also respond to these medications.

Essential tremor is often mistaken for Parkinson's disease. Essential tremor can be somewhat asymmetric and can sometimes be seen with the arms in a position of rest. For this reason we do not make a diagnosis of Parkinson's disease in a patient who only has tremor, although a classic parkinsonian rest tremor does suggest the possibility that other cardinal features will develop over time. A five-year history of bilateral upper extremity tremor without the emergence of bradykinesia or rigidity suggests a diagnosis of essential tremor rather than Parkinson's disease.

WILSON'S DISEASE is a disorder of copper metabolism transmitted by autosomal recessive inheritance[18]. The responsible gene has been mapped to the long arm of chromosome 13. Wilson's disease is a disease of children, adolescents and young adults. Symptoms rarely occur before age 6 or after age 40. In children, hepatobiliary symptoms predominate whereas in adolescents and young adults neuropsychiatric symptoms are the rule. The exact etiology is unknown but results in a positive copper balance. Free copper deposits in the liver and brain, leading to cirrhosis and neuropsychiatric features. The disease is associated with low levels of ceruloplasmin, a serum protein responsible for binding copper, increased liver copper concentration, and increased urinary copper excretion. Patients may present with tremor (often of a "wing-beating" variety), dysarthria, rigidity, bradykinesia, dystonia and psychiatric disturbances.

A pathognomonic feature of the neuropsychiatric form of the disease is the presence of Kayser-Fleischer rings, a brownish discoloration of the peripheral cornea seen on slit lamp examination of the eyes. Any young

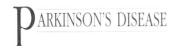

patient presenting with an unexplained tremor, parkinsonism or abnormal movements should receive a screening evaluation for Wilson's disease. This includes a serum ceruloplasmin level determination, measurement of urinary copper, and an ophthalmologic examination. Treatment includes decreasing the amount of copper in the diet, as well as use of a copper chelator, such as D-penicillamine. Wilson's disease is one of the few potentially devastating genetic diseases for which there are effective medical therapies. A high index of suspicion is required to diagnose this treatable disorder.

HALLERVORDEN-SPATZ SYNDROME is a disease of the young, from infancy to young adulthood. Most cases are thought to be transmitted by autosomal recessive inheritance. Patients present with extrapyramidal symptoms including dystonia, rigidity, choreoathetosis and tremor, corticospinal tract signs, and dementia. The clinical course is progressive, leading to death. Abnormal accumulation of iron has been found in the GP and SNr of affected individuals. This massive accumulation of iron often produces prominent signal hypointensity in the GP and SNr on high field strength T2-weighted MRI. There is currently no effective treatment.

NEUROACANTHOCYTOSIS is characterized clinically by adult onset, progressive orofacial dyskinesia, chorea and dystonia of the limbs, and a predominantly motor polyneuropathy with amyotrophy[19]. Additional signs can include seizures, parkinsonism, areflexia, and variable psychiatric disturbances with or without dementia. Some patients experience a progressive akinetic-rigid syndrome that gradually replaces the hyperkinetic features[20]. It is usually transmitted by autosomal recessive inheritance although autosomal dominant, x-linked and sporadic cases have also been reported.

Characteristic laboratory findings include increased levels of serum creatinine kinase and acanthocytes, erythrocytes with irregular spines projecting from the cell surface, presumably caused by a defect in membrane lipids. Pathology findings include atrophy of the caudate nuclei and putamena, and occasionally of the globi pallidi. Anterior horn cell loss may be present as well as chronic axonal neuropathy with demyelination[21]. Treatment is limited to symptomatic therapy with neuroleptics for chorea and anticonvulsants for seizures. Patients with bradykinesia or rigidity may respond to dopaminergic therapy.

HUNTINGTON'S DISEASE is a degenerative, autosomal-dominant disorder characterized by chorea, personality changes, and dementia [22]. Onset usually occurs in middle age, although some cases begin in childhood or adolescence [23]. Huntington's disease is caused by an increased number of trinucleotide (CAG) repeats in the gene on the short arm of chromosome 4 [24]. The worldwide prevalence is 5-10 per 100,000. There is no therapy known to slow the progression of the disease and death commonly occurs 15-20 years after onset of symptoms.

Family members may notice that an affected patient has become short-tempered and depressed. He or she may be unable to sit still for any period of time, and may develop involuntary movements of the limbs, with decreased ocular saccades. Eventually, involuntary choreiform movements emerge, along with dementia. Atrophy of the caudate and putamen may be seen on imaging studies. Suicide is fairly common if depression is present, and patients are usually confined to a nursing home in the later stages. Therapy is limited to symptomatic treatment using antidepressants for depression and neuroleptics when necessary to control chorea [25]. Neuroleptics reduce chorea but often at the expense of side-effects including apathy, sedation, akathisia, and parkinsonism. They should be reserved for those patients in whom chorea impairs function or self-care.

Five to ten percent of patients have juvenile Huntington's disease with onset before age twenty. Juvenile Huntington's disease is usually manifest by parkinsonian symptoms including bradykinesia, rigidity, and sometimes tremor. Dystonia and impaired eye movements may predominate and patients may have seizures. Ninety percent of juvenile Huntington's disease patients inherit the gene from an affected father, due to the large increase in the number of triplet repeats that can occur during spermatogenesis. Bradykinesia and rigidity may improve with levodopa therapy.

What are the "atypical parkinsonisms"?

The atypical parkinsonisms are a group of adult-onset progressive neurologic disorders that are characterized by bradykinesia and rigidity clinically and more widespread neuronal degeneration than Parkinson's disease histologically. The atypical parkinsonisms include progressive supranuclear palsy, corticobasal degeneration, and the multiple system atrophies. The multiple system atrophies are a group of closely related disorders that include degeneration in the extrapyramidal, pyramidal, autonomic and cerebellar systems.

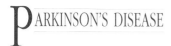

How can I clinically recognize the atypical parkinsonisms?

In contrast to Parkinson's disease, the atypical parkinsonisms are generally symmetric, lack resting tremor, and respond little, if at all, to dopaminergic medications. There is usually early speech and balance impairment, and rigidity may be greater in the neck than the extremities. Some of the atypical parkinsonisms are associated with characteristic clinical signs that aid in their identification. The most important diagnostic distinction is between Parkinson's disease, which responds well to medical therapy, and the atypical parkinsonisms that do not.

What is progressive supranuclear palsy?

Progressive supranuclear palsy (PSP) is one of the atypical parkinsonisms or "parkinson plus" syndromes. It was originally described by Steele, Richardson, and Olszewski[26], and has a prevalence of approximately 7/100,000 individuals over age 55[27]. PSP has a later mean age of onset than Parkinson's disease, and most patients are in their sixties or seventies.

PSP is marked by bradykinesia and rigidity, postural instability, dysarthria, gait disturbances, and speech and swallowing difficulty[28]. Tremor is unusual. The characteristic clinical sign of PSP is a supranuclear gaze palsy. This refers to the fact that the patient is unable to voluntarily move in the eyes, but the eyes move normally in response to passive head movements (oculocephalic testing). This finding implies that the difficulty must be above the nuclei that control voluntary eye movements, and hence it is called supranuclear palsy. Downgaze is first affected followed by upgaze and later horizontal gaze. Slow saccade velocity may precede limitations of eye movements[28].

Some patients may complain of difficulty looking down, or note blurred vision but many have no visual complaints. Blink rate is markedly reduced and there may be "ocular stare" with the upper eyelids resting above the irises. Some patients exhibit neck extension rather than the stooped posture of Parkinson's disease. When turning, patients may cross their feet rather than turning "en bloc" as do Parkinson's disease patients. Falling due to imbalance occurs relatively early, often within a year or two of symptom onset. Blepharospasm and other focal dystonias are not unusual[29]. Dementia similar to that seen in patients with frontal lobe dysfunction is relatively common, particularly later in the disease[30]. On pathology examination, neuronal degeneration is present in the pallidum, subthalamic nucleus, and other areas. Lewy bodies are absent.

What are the multiple-system atrophies?

The multiple-system atrophies (MSAs) include striatonigral degeneration, Shy-Drager syndrome, and olivopontocerebellar atrophy[31,32]. Neuronal degeneration is much more widespread than in Parkinson's disease, and may include the striatum, substantia nigra, olives, pons, cerebellum, and spinal cord[32]. Lewy bodies are absent. Clinical symptoms of basal ganglia dysfunction, as well as cerebellar and autonomic dysfunction may be present. The early onset of frequent falling, coupled with cerebellar, pyramidal, or autonomic dysfunction usually suggests a diagnosis of MSA. Resting tremor is unusual but may be seen in some cases. Speech is more severely affected in MSA than in Parkinson's disease, and patients often develop early and dramatic hypophonia. Abnormal eye movements consisting of slow saccades or impaired convergence may be present. Myoclonic jerks may also occur. Response to dopaminergic therapy is poor and treatment consists of symptomatic and supportive care.

What is Shy-Drager syndrome?

Shy-Drager syndrome is an atypical parkinsonism characterized by prominent autonomic dysfunction. Clinical features of autonomic dysfunction may include orthostatic hypotension (or syncope), impotence, urinary incontinence and sweating abnormalities. Vocal cord paralysis, speech disturbances, sleep apnea, and psychiatric changes may also occur.

G. Milton Shy and Glenn Drager originally described a group of patients with orthostatic hypotension, urinary incontinence, loss of sweating, ocular palsies, iris atrophy, rigidity, impotence, and wasting of distal musculature with EMG findings suggestive of anterior horn cell involvement[33]. The disorder most commonly affects patients in their 50s to 70s, and is more common in men. Impotence is a common early manifestation in men, while lightheadedness is often the first noticed feature in women. The disease is progressive, and ultimately leads to death.

On pathology, marked gliosis is seen in the intermediolateral column of the spinal cord with changes noted in sympathetic ganglia. Cell degeneration is also seen in the inferior olivary nucleus, dorsal vagus nucleus, and substantia nigra pars compacta. Abnormalities may be seen in the cerebellum, Edinger-Westphal nucleus, oculomotor nucleus, and caudate nucleus. Noradrenergic neurons of brain and sympathetic ganglia are affected, with marked loss of tyrosine hydroxylase activity in the locus ceruleus. Dopamine-b-hydroxylase activity has also been found to be diminished in sympathetic ganglia [34].

Dopaminergic medications are usually not of benefit and may worsen symptoms of orthostasis [35]. Symptomatic therapy for orthostatic hypotension may be helpful.

What is olivopontocerebellar atrophy?

Olivopontocerebellar atrophy (OPCA) is characterized by parkinsonism and cerebellar dysfunction [36]. The disease may occur by autosomal dominant inheritance or sporadically, and may affect individuals from infancy through the sixth decade. Patients may present with gait ataxia, extrapyramidal and pyramidal signs, and sphincter disturbances. Familial cases usually begin at a younger age, progress more slowly, and exhibit less autonomic failure than sporadic cases.

Cerebellar abnormalities are usually the presenting feature of dominantly inherited forms of OPCA. Parkinsonian symptoms may be early or late manifestations [37]. Speech difficulties, swallowing impairment, dementia, and visual disturbances may also occur. Response to dopaminergic therapy is usually poor. Neuronal degeneration occurs in the pons, inferior olives, and cerebellar cortex as well as the substantia nigra, pyramidal tracts, and thalamus [38]. CT and MRI typically show cerebellar atrophy, with widened cerebellopontine cisterns [39].

What is striatonigral degeneration?

Striatonigral degeneration [40] is an adult-onset progressive, symmetric, bradykinetic-rigid disorder characterized by early falling, speech and swallowing difficulties. Hyperreflexia and sleep apnea may be present. Resting tremor is much less common than in Parkinson's disease, and response to dopaminergic therapy is poor. Age at onset is comparable to that of Parkinson's disease, but progression of disability is much more rapid. On pathology, neuronal loss is found in the striatum, with widespread changes also noted elsewhere [41]. Cell loss is also seen in the substantia nigra, but Lewy bodies are rare.

What is corticobasal ganglionic degeneration?

Corticobasal ganglionic degeneration is a progressive, adult-onset bradykinetic-rigid syndrome characterized by the presence of both parkinsonism and cortical dysfunction. In contrast to other atypical parkinsonisms, there is often marked asymmetry. Parkinsonian features include bradykinesia and asymmetric limb rigidity. Cortical features include apraxia and cortical sensory loss [42,43]. Patients may have involuntary mirror movements or levitation of an arm ("alien-limb" phenomenon). Associated features include postural instability, hyperreflexia, focal reflex myoclonus, and apraxia of eye movement. On pathology the disease is characterized by asymmetric atrophy of the frontal and parietal lobes, and substantia nigra with neuronal achromasia [44]. There is no treatment known to be effective for this disorder. Injections of botulinum toxin are sometimes useful to reduce marked rigidity in an arm or hand but do not improve limb function.

What is Lewy body disease?

Lewy body disease is an atypical parkinsonism characterized by dementia, and autonomic abnormalities. It is marked pathologically by cortical and brainstem Lewy bodies [45,46]. Symptoms include dementia often with fluctuations in cognitive state, hallucinations, and depression. Dementia usually occurs early in the disease, and parkinsonian features follow. Dysphasia and agnosia may also occur. On pathology, Lewy bodies are found in the cortex, limbus, hypothalamus, and brainstem nuclei. Dopamine medications may readily induce or worsen hallucinations.

CHAPTER 4

CLINICAL FEATURES OF PARKINSON'S DISEASE

What are the cardinal features of Parkinson's disease?

The four cardinal signs of Parkinson's disease are resting tremor, rigidity, bradykinesia, and postural instability. Tremor is the oscillation of a body part about a joint and is commonly observed as "shaking back and forth." Rigidity refers to increased resistance (stiffness) when a joint is passively flexed and extended. Bradykinesia means slowness of movement. It also encompasses decreased spontaneous movements and decreased amplitude of movement.

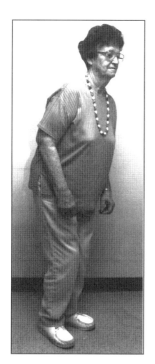

Postural instability refers to imbalance and in contrast to the first three cardinal features does not emerge until late in the disease. The most common initial finding is an asymmetric resting tremor although about twenty percent of patients first experience clumsiness of a hand[1].

What other clinical features are associated with Parkinson's disease?

Patients with early Parkinson's disease often notice difficulty with fine coordinated movements and daily tasks become more difficult. There may be more difficulty buttoning shirts, combing one's hair, or playing golf. The first-affected arm may not swing fully when walking, and the foot on the same side may scuff or drag along the floor. Handwriting may become small (micrographia) and cramped. Family members may notice decreased facial expression (masked face). Speech may become soft (hypophonia) and monotonal. Axial posture becomes progressively flexed and strides are shortened (figure 4-1), thereby causing

Figure 4-1. *Characteristic flexed posture of a patient with Parkinson's disease. (used with permission)*

a "shuffling" gait. The patient may eventually notice drooling and have difficulty swallowing foods.

Pain may occur in an affected limb, sometimes leading to an erroneous diagnosis of arthritis or bursitis. Often this aching pain involves a large muscle group on one side of the body, commonly the calf. This can be accompanied by movement (dystonia) in the leg, with the foot or toes turning down or in. Patients may notice a change in the taste of food caused by a lack of smell (anosmia). Depression can occur at any time throughout the disease. Symptoms of autonomic dysfunction include constipation, urinary frequency, sweating abnormalities, dermatitis, and sexual dysfunction. Patients may also experience sleep disturbances. Dementia may emerge over many years.

How does one make the diagnosis of Parkinson's disease?

The best clinical predictors of a pathology diagnosis of Parkinson's disease are:

a. asymmetry of onset
b. presence of resting tremor
c. good response to dopamine medication therapy.

The clinical diagnosis of Parkinson's disease is made by evaluation of the patient's history, neurologic examination, and response to dopamine replacement therapy. There are no blood tests that make the diagnosis and brain CT and MRI are typically unrevealing.

The following categories have been proposed for a clinical diagnosis of idiopathic Parkinson's disease [2]:

1. It is POSSIBLE that the patient has Parkinson's disease if one of the following is present: tremor (either resting or postural), rigidity, or bradykinesia.

2. It is PROBABLE that the patient has Parkinson's disease if two of the major features (resting tremor, rigidity, bradykinesia, or postural instability) are present, or if resting tremor, rigidity, or bradykinesia are asymmetric.

3. It is DEFINITE that the patient has Parkinson's disease if three of the major features are present, or if two of the features are present with one of them presenting asymmetrically.

Causes of secondary parkinsonism are excluded before a diagnosis of idiopathic Parkinson's disease is made (see chapter 3). These include medications, cerebrovascular disease, toxins, infections, and metabolic abnormalities. Other degenerative disorders (Creutzfeld-Jacob disease, Gerstmann-Straussler syndrome, Wilson's disease, Huntington's disease, neuroacanthocytosis), and conditions (normal pressure hydrocephalus) must also be excluded.

How reliable is a diagnosis of Parkinson's disease?

Two clinical-pathological studies found that 25% of patients diagnosed by neurologists with PD during life actually had other diagnoses based on autopsy findings. Autopsy evaluations in these patients were consistent with striatonigral degeneration, progressive supranuclear palsy, multi-infarct dementia, and Alzheimer's disease [3-5]. Interestingly, two-thirds of misdiagnosed patients reported a good to excellent response to levodopa, although the true extent of their response is not known.

It is very important to determine if parkinsonian symptoms including tremor, rigidity and bradykinesia truly improve with levodopa therapy. A meaningful (>50%) and sustained improvement in parkinsonian signs is thought to be a strong indicator of a pathology diagnosis of PD, but non-specific, unsustained or slight improvement is not. Fortunately, misdiagnosis based on clinical presentation and response to medication rarely causes a missed opportunity for improvement, as most mimickers of PD do not respond to any treatment. The exception to this is Wilson's disease (see chapter 3) which does require treatment to avoid irreversible damage.

What are the clinical characteristics of the tremor of Parkinson's disease?

Resting tremor is the most common presenting feature of Parkinson's disease, affecting almost seventy percent of patients [1]. It may be present in one or more limbs and is usually asymmetric. Tremor is typically present when the limb is at rest, but may also be seen with the limb in a position of postural maintenance (e.g., with the arms outstretched).

The characteristic tremor is a "pill-rolling" movement of the fingers or flexion/extension of the fingers or wrist. The frequency of the tremor is usually four to five cycles per second. The amplitude is quite variable and may change from minute to minute. The amplitude commonly increases in periods of stress such as when the patient is asked to perform a cognitive task. Like most tremors, it disappears during sleep. The resting tremor of Parkinson's disease can be difficult to treat because of its variable response to medication therapy.

What is akinesia?

Akinesia literally means "lack of movement". In clinical use, it is synonymous with bradykinesia. These terms refer to slowness in the initiation and execution of movement. Parkinson's disease patients have longer reaction times coupled with an element of inattention that adds to their "slowness". This difficulty of movement is often described as the most disabling feature of the disease.

How does akinesia differ from akathisia?

Akathisia refers to a compulsion to move about and is commonly expressed as an inability to remain seated[6]. The initial stages of akathisia involve an inner feeling of restlessness, followed by the need to move. Unlike levodopa-induced dyskinesia, which is comprised of involuntary choreiform (random twisting, turning) movements, akathisia does not involve abnormal types of movement but rather an increased quantity of normal movements. Patients may march in place, pace back and forth, or perform repetitive movements of the limbs. Its exact etiology is unknown but is probably related to insufficient dopamine innervation. It is somewhat uncommon in Parkinson's disease, but is much more common in psychiatric patients.

In psychiatric patients, akathisia is commonly induced by anti-psychotic medications. In this setting, akathisia may be difficult to differentiate from the restlessness of psychotic agitation. Treatment of akathisia involves reduction of anti-dopaminergic medication, or the possible use of anticholinergics, antihistamines, or dopaminergic medications. Some studies have found beta-blockers to be helpful[5].

How do young and old onset Parkinson's disease patients differ?

Five to ten percent of Parkinson's disease patients experience onset of symptoms before age forty[7]. Patients who develop PD under age 21 are considered "juvenile PD" patients, while those who develop the disease from age 21 through 40 are said to have "young onset PD (YOPD)". The prevalence of PD in patients under age 40 is generally estimated at 0-0.8 per 100,000 [3-5,8,9], although some studies found a prevalence rate as high as 4.7/100,000 [10,11].

Schrag et al. examined 139 YOPD patients, and found that all developed motor fluctuations and dyskinesia by 10 years post-diagnosis. Mortality risk was double that of the normal population. The median survival was 27 years for PD patients with disease onset from 36-39 years, and 35 years for patients with disease onset from 22-35 years. Cognitive impairment occurred in only 19% of patients [9].

A young patient who presents with parkinsonian features warrants a careful screen to rule out secondary causes of parkinsonism, especially those that are potentially treatable, such as Wilson's disease. Young onset Parkinson's disease patients are usually quite responsive to dopamine replacement therapy, have less dementia, and more readily develop levodopa-induced dyskinesias than their older counterparts [12]. Older patients are more likely to develop progressive bradykinesia that responds only partially to levodopa, and more likely to develop dementia.

How common are neuropsychiatric disturbances in Parkinson's disease?

In one sample of 139 PD patients in Norway, at least one "psychiatric" symptom was reported in 61% of patients. The most common psychiatric manifestations are depression (38%) and hallucinations (27%). Less common symptoms are euphoria and disinhibition [13]. Other studies have reported prevalence rates of psychosis in PD ranging from 6% to 40%, including visual hallucinations, delusions, dysphoria, mania, delirium, and abnormal sexual behavior [14-17].

What is the most common form of psychosis in Parkinson's disease?

Patients may develop hallucinations, particularly as a side effect of dopamine medications. Typically these are visual hallucinations in which patients see people or animals.

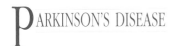

What are the risk factors for developing psychosis in Parkinson's disease?

Juncos et al. found that the most significant risk factors for developing psychosis in PD are the presence of dementia, protracted sleep disturbances, and nighttime use of long-acting dopamine medications[14].

How common is dementia in Parkinson's disease?

Dementia is defined as a loss of intellectual abilities of sufficient severity to interfere with social or occupational functioning[18]. The loss of intellectual function almost always involves memory impairment, and may be associated with personality changes, impaired judgment, and difficulty with abstract thinking. Dementia is fairly common in Parkinson's disease. Reported prevalence rates range from 10% to 80%[19], but actual rates are probably closer to 15% to 30%[20]. Dementia usually emerges late in the course of PD, often after eight to ten years.

What causes dementia in Parkinson's disease?

The presence of dementia in PD is highly correlated with the presence of Lewy bodies staining for alpha-synuclein in the cortex[21]. This suggests that the same disease process that is causing loss of nigrostriatal dopamine neurons is occurring in the cortex of patients with dementia. Why this occurs in some PD cases but not others is not known. Alzheimer's disease pathology is found in only a small minority of demented PD patients.

Short-term memory may be specifically affected in patients with Parkinson's disease, while immediate recall and long term memory remain fairly intact[22]. There may be increased processing time with longer response latencies. Visuospatial function may also be impaired.

Which patients with Parkinson's disease are at the highest risk to develop dementia?

One study found that PD patients who developed dementia were older at disease onset and had a longer duration of disease[9]. Dementia may also be related to disease subtype. In a series of 155 PD patients, 8% had severe dementia. Almost half of demented PD patients suffered from the akinetic-rigid form of the disease (slowness and stiffness without tremor), whereas only 19% of non-demented patients had the akinetic-rigid form[9,11].

How common is depression in Parkinson's disease patients?

Depression is the most commonly encountered "psychiatric" symptom in Parkinson's disease. As many as 40 to 50% of patients are affected by mood changes [23]. Depression in Parkinson's disease is more commonly associated with dysphoria and sadness, rather than self-blame or guilt [24]. It can occur at any time during the course of the disease and may emerge prior to motor symptoms. Several studies have reported a greater incidence of depression in female patients, but this remains controversial.

What causes depression in Parkinson's disease?

Depression in Parkinson's disease probably has both endogenous and reactive components. Several studies have found that depressed PD patients have lower levels of CSF 5-HIAA, the major metabolite of serotonin, as occurs in non-parkinsonian patients diagnosed with major depression [24]. Antidepressants are usually effective in treating depression associated with Parkinson's disease.

What are the autonomic disturbances associated with Parkinson's disease?

Autonomic dysfunction is an important cause of non-motor features of Parkinson's disease. James Parkinson described some of these symptoms in his original essay. Autonomic abnormalities may include:

- orthostatic hypotension
  (lightheadedness due to a drop in blood pressure upon standing)
- constipation
- gastrointestinal disorders
  (decreased gastric emptying, swallowing difficulties)
- decreased salivation
- sphincter dysfunction
- impotence
- heat intolerance
- increased sweating
- livedo reticularis
  (skin discoloration)
- seborrhea.

As many as 70 to 80% of Parkinson's disease patients experience some degree of autonomic dysfunction [25]. Many patients develop a loss of variation in heart rate interval (R-R) in response to postural changes [26]. This is indicative of parasympathetic system dysfunction. Lewy bodies have been found in the lateral hypothalamus in Parkinson's disease patients, an

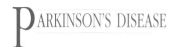

area important to regulation of the parasympathetic system [27]. Autonomic dysfunction may also be caused by abnormalities in the sympathetic ganglia. Treatment of autonomic dysfunction is symptomatic.

Is sleepiness a symptom of Parkinson's disease?

Abnormal sleepiness occurs in about 50% of PD patients [28]. Increased awareness regarding sleepiness in PD followed the report of Frucht et al. describing episodes of sudden-onset, irresistible sleep ("sleep attacks") leading to motor vehicle accidents in eight patients taking dopamine agonist medications [29]. It is now clear that any of the dopamine medications can potentially cause daytime sleepiness or episodes of unintended sleep, although somnolence is a more common side effect of dopamine agonists than levodopa [28,30,31]. In addition, sleep disorders are common in PD and the disease itself also causes sleepiness.

One way to evaluate sleepiness is to determine the time to fall asleep during nap opportunities, a technique known as multiple sleep latency testing (MSLT). Using this methodology, Rye et al. found that 37% of PD patients fell asleep in less than five minutes on average, consistent with pathological sleepiness [32]. Moreover, patients who were not taking any dopamine medications were as sleepy as patients on dopamine medications. This suggests that Parkinson's disease itself causes sleepiness.

What sleep disorders occur in Parkinson's disease?

Several sleep disorders can be seen in Parkinson's disease including REM behavior disorder (RBD), restless legs syndrome (RLS), and sleep apnea.

RBD is characterized by lack of muscle atonia during REM sleep leading to "acting out of dreams", including sleep talking, shouting, and intense, sometimes violent movements. RBD has been reported in up to 50% of PD patients and can precede the clinical onset of Parkinson's disease by several years [33,34].

Restless legs syndrome occurs in approximately 20% of PD patients [28]. Individuals with this disorder experience uncomfortable sensations in the legs that are worse at night and when lying in bed. The sensations are variably described as a creepy crawly sensation, or "pepsi cola in the veins". These sensations are temporarily reduced or improved when the patient moves his legs. Many RLS patients find the sensations so uncomfortable that they can't sleep and end up walking around at night to relieve them.

Obstructive sleep apnea also occurs in about 20% of PD patients [35]. In this disorder, airflow during sleep is intermittently absent or reduced despite respiratory effort. In the general population, patients with sleep apnea are commonly stocky or obese, snore during sleep, and do not feel refreshed in the morning. Whether these predictors apply to sleep apnea in PD is not yet known. Treatment usually consists of wearing an airflow mask (continuous positive airway pressure, CPAP) although many patients find it uncomfortable.

What other sleep disturbances do Parkinson's disease patients experience? A common complaint of Parkinson's disease patients is the inability to get a full night of restful sleep. Patients describe both an inability to fall asleep and numerous nighttime awakenings. Patients may have difficulty falling asleep due to depression or persistent tremor. Early awakenings may be caused by a reemergence of symptoms at night as daytime medications wear off. Reemergence of tremor may turn a light arousal into a complete awakening. Rigidity and akinesia can make it impossible to turn over in bed. Some patients develop a reversal of sleep-wake patterns and may nap excessively during the day and remain awake at night.

Sleep difficulties may be related to abnormalities in arousal mechanisms due to autonomic nervous system dysfunction [36]. In addition, endogenous levels of serotonin, important for slow wave sleep, are decreased in Parkinson's disease [37]. Some patients may benefit from the judicious use of sleeping medications.

What are the stages of Parkinson's disease?

One way to describe the severity of Parkinson's disease is the Hoehn and Yahr scale, developed by Margaret Hoehn and Melvin Yahr in the 1960s [7]. This scale describes five "stages" of Parkinson's disease. The scale reflects worsening disease severity but is not a linear indicator of disease progression [38].

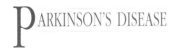

Stage I: Unilateral features of Parkinson's disease, including the major features of tremor, rigidity, or bradykinesia.

Stage II: Bilateral features mentioned above, along with possible speech abnormalities, decreased posture, and abnormal gait.

Stage III: Worsening bilateral features of Parkinson's disease, along with balance difficulties. Patients are still able to function independently.

Stage IV: Patients are unable to live alone or independently.

Stage V: Patients need wheelchair assistance, or are unable to get out of bed.

Disease corresponding to stages IV and V was found in 37% and 42% of patients with disease duration of 10 and 15 years, respectively [38]. However, Hoehn and Yahr also found considerable variability; 34% of patients with a disease duration of 10 years or longer were still in stages I or II, reflecting heterogeneity of the disease [38,39].

How are the signs and symptoms of Parkinson's disease assessed in research studies?

The most commonly employed research scale is the "Unified Parkinson's Disease Rating Scale (UPDRS)". Individual features are graded on a 0 to 4 scale. Features that are scored include facial expression, voice, tremor, rigidity, bradykinesia, gait, and balance. The individual scores can be summed to arrive at subset scores for mentation, activities of daily living, and motor function, as well as a total score [40].

What other systems are used to describe Parkinson's disease severity? We find it very helpful to use a classification system based on medications and clinical response. The classes provide a shorthand description and often correspond with entry criteria for clinical trials. They reflect key clinical information that tends to guide treatment decisions.

CLINICAL CLASSIFICATION OF PARKINSON'S DISEASE PATIENTS

Class 1:
Patient is not on any antiparkinsonian medications ("de novo").

Class 2:
Patient is on antiparkinsonian medication but not levodopa.

Class 3:
Patient is on levodopa and experiencing a stable response.

Class 4:
Patient is on levodopa and experiencing motor fluctuations without dyskinesia.

Class 5:
Patient is on levodopa and experiencing motor fluctuations and dyskinesia.

CHAPTER 5

COMPLICATIONS OF LONG TERM THERAPY IN PD AND THE CONTINUOUS DOPAMINERGIC STIMULATION HYPOTHESIS

Levodopa, the precursor to dopamine, has been considered the "gold standard" of treatment for PD for many years because it provides the greatest antiparkinsonian efficacy with the fewest short term side-effects. However, its use is complicated by the development of long term side-effects, specifically motor fluctuations and dyskinesias. The development of these long term complications is thought to be due to a combination of disease progression and levodopa's short half-life.

Levodopa is usually administered with a peripheral decarboxylase inhibitor (PDI) such as carbidopa that reduces levodopa's metabolism in the blood and decreases nausea. The half-life of levodopa when administered with carbidopa is approximately 90 minutes. This means that levodopa is mostly cleared from the blood within 4-6 hours after administration.

What is the usual course of treated Parkinson's disease?

Patients usually experience good control of parkinsonian features when symptomatic therapy is first introduced. This "honeymoon" period is maintained for approximately three to five years into levodopa therapy [1,2]. Although levodopa has a short serum (blood) half-life, patients initially experience a stable response through the day (figure 5-1). This is presumably due to the ability of remaining nigrostriatal neurons to generate dopamine from absorbed levodopa, store it intraneuronally and slowly release it into the synaptic cleft in a relatively normal fashion. Because there are 60-80% fewer dopamine neurons, the amount of dopamine released from each neuron is increased (increased dopamine turnover) in order to approximate the normal state.

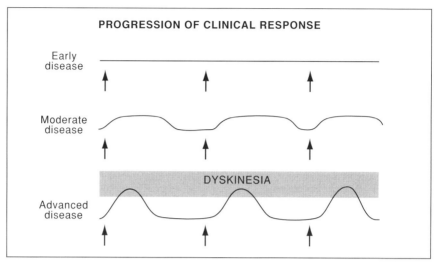

Figure 5-1. *Progression of clinical response in Parkinson's disease. Despite the short half-life of levodopa/PDI, patients with early disease experience a sustained response through the day. As the disease progresses, patients begin to notice "wearing-off" fluctuations such that the benefit of levodopa/PDI wears off after a few hours. Ultimately, clinical response fluctuates more and more closely in association with peripheral levodopa and patients develop choreiform dyskinesia when dopamine peaks. Arrows indicate times of levodopa/PDI administration.*

Despite levodopa therapy, disability continues to progress over time [3]. This may be due to inadequate dopamine stimulation or degeneration of neurons downstream to dopamine receptors. Over the years there is a tendency to administer increasing amounts of dopaminergic medication in order to minimize functional disability.

Motor fluctuations begin to emerge as early as one to two years after initiation of levodopa therapy. Between approximately four and eight years, many patients experience motor fluctuations and dyskinesia that cause clinical disability. Patients begin to notice that whereas they used to be able to take standard levodopa/PDI three or four times a day and still maintain a stable response, the benefit now lasts a few hours and then wears off. Patients may initially notice a short duration levodopa response of four to five hours. Over the next few years, the short duration response becomes more fleeting and benefit lasts only two to three hours. Over time, clinical status more and more closely fluctuates in concert with peripheral levodopa concentration [4]. Presumably, this is because as neuronal degeneration progresses, the capacity for surviving neurons to effectively store levodopa-derived dopamine diminishes.

During this time, many patients also develop peak-dose dyskinesias consisting of twisting, turning (choreiform) movements that occur when central (brain) dopamine levels are peaking[5,6]. This marks an important milestone in the treatment of Parkinson's disease because it limits the amount of dopaminergic therapy that can be provided. At this point, higher doses of dopaminergic therapy are likely to increase peak-dose dyskinesia. This "hypersensitivity" may result from exposing post-synaptic receptors to rapidly fluctuating levodopa-derived dopamine levels[4].

From five to ten years into symptomatic therapy, much of the management of Parkinson's disease centers on titrating therapy to maximize ON time without dyskinesia. Too much dopaminergic therapy exacerbates peak-dose dyskinesias and too little dopaminergic therapy fails to bring about sufficient benefit. Despite optimal titration, many patients eight or more years into symptomatic therapy suffer with troublesome or disabling motor fluctuations and dyskinesia.

Some patients develop dementia as the disease progresses. As antiparkinsonian therapy can worsen confusion and hallucinations, the presence of cognitive dysfunction can also limit administration of medication to improve motor symptoms.

By ten to twelve years or more, many patients have developed balance difficulty. This is another important milestone. True balance difficulty (postural imbalance) is not improved by any current antiparkinsonian therapy. Patients are then at risk for morbidity and mortality from falls. Immobility may place a patient at increased risk for infections and swallowing difficulty may increase the risk of aspiration and malnutrition. The cause of death in Parkinson's disease is often related to infection, injuries due to falls or other medical conditions such as stroke or heart attack.

Individual progression varies greatly. Some patients maintain relatively good function fifteen years into the disease and others experience meaningful disability within a few years.

What are the complications of long term levodopa therapy in Parkinson's disease?

The complications of long term therapy for Parkinson's disease include motor fluctuations and dyskinesia. Motor fluctuations consist of variations in clinical

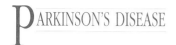

status that occurs over the course of a day. Dyskinesia refers to abnormal involuntary movements occurring in association with medication therapy.

What are the different types of motor fluctuations?

Wearing-off fluctuations are relatively predictable variations in motor function temporally associated with the timing of levodopa ingestion. After several years of stable response through the day, many patients experience benefit for only a few hours following levodopa ingestion. This is followed by a loss of benefit, or wearing-off. Symptom control can be regained by taking the next levodopa dose. In contrast, on-off fluctuations are rapid transitions (over seconds) between the on and off states, seemingly unrelated to the timing of medication ingestion.

What are the ON and OFF states?

ON and OFF states can be identified in patients with motor fluctuations. ON refers to a patient's clinical status when medication is providing symptomatic benefit with regard to mobility, bradykinesia, and rigidity. OFF refers to a patient's status when symptomatic benefit has been lost over the preceding minutes or hours. Some patients also experience an intermediate state as re-emergence of tremor may precede loss of benefit for mobility, bradykinesia and rigidity.

Will my patient recognize motor fluctuations?

Patients with a stable response commonly report that they are unsure if they are experiencing motor fluctuations. In contrast, patients with motor fluctuations can usually identify these fluctuations without difficulty.

Does wearing off effect other symptoms?

Although wearing off was first defined as a wearing off of benefit regarding motor symptoms, many patients also describe re-emergence of non-motor symptoms when levodopa wears off. These can include mood changes such as depression or anxiety, autonomic symptoms such as sweating, or cognitive changes such as cloudiness or slowing of thinking.

Is a worsening of tremor during periods of stress a type of motor fluctuation?

No. Patients commonly experience a transient increase in tremor (or dyskinesia) when emotionally activated. This phenomenon is not related to the pharmacokinetics of levodopa. Its cause is poorly understood.

What are the types of dyskinesia that occur in Parkinson's disease?

Involuntary abnormal movements associated with medication intake are categorized by the type of movement and the phase of the dosing cycle in which they occur. The three most common types of dyskinesia in Parkinson's disease are peak-dose dyskinesia, wearing-off dystonia, and diphasic dystonia/dyskinesia. They are relatively specific to Parkinson's disease and often worse on the side of the body most affected. They usually emerge in patients who have had a good response to levodopa and the incidence is highest in young-onset patients[6].

Peak-dose dyskinesias are most common. They occur at the peak of the dosing cycle, when levodopa-derived dopamine is highest. They consist of choreiform, non-patterned, twisting, turning movements usually seen in the extremities, trunk, and head. They diminish when the levodopa dose is reduced and increase when the levodopa dose is raised.

Wearing-off dystonia occurs in association with low or falling dopamine levels[7]. It commonly occurs at night or in the morning prior to the first levodopa dose. It consists of involuntary, sustained muscle contractions and commonly occurs in the lower extremities causing foot inversion or plantar flexion. The dystonia may be associated with pain, particularly in the calf. It may respond to more sustained dopaminergic stimulation as provided by dopamine agonists, extended release levodopa/carbidopa, or levodopa/carbidopa plusentacapone.

Diphasic dystonia/dyskinesia is relatively uncommon and occurs both when a patient is turning on and when wearing off. It was originally called D-I-D dystonia/dyskinesia, indicating dystonia/dyskinesia was followed by improvement and then a return of dystonia/dyskinesia within a single dosing cycle[5]. It is often manifest as a combination of dystonia and chorea, and typically affects the lower extremities. Diphasic dyskinesia can

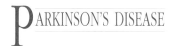

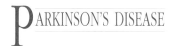

be difficult to treat but usually an attempt is made to increase and smooth dopaminergic stimulation. D-I-D dyskinesia is often improved by deep brain stimulation of the globus pallidus or subthalamic nucleus (see surgery chapter).

It can usually be assumed that chorea in the setting of treated Parkinson's disease represents peak-dose dyskinesia until proven otherwise because it is so common. The unqualified term dyskinesia in the context of Parkinson's disease usually refers to peak-dose dyskinesia.

How common are the long term complications?

More than 50% of patients treated five years or longer may have motor fluctuations and dyskinesia [8]. Approximately 90% of patients develop motor fluctuations and dyskinesia by 15 years of disease.

Are these long term complications caused by levodopa?

Normal individuals do not appear to develop motor fluctuations or dyskinesia if administered levodopa. The emergence of long term complications probably occurs as a result of the combination of disease progression and levodopa administration.

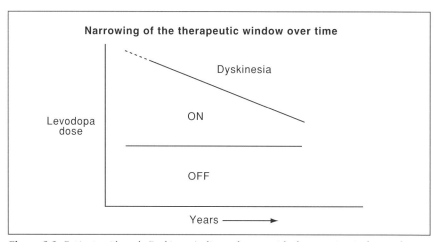

Figure 5-2. *Patients with early Parkinson's disease have a wide therapeutic window and respond well to a wide range of levodopa dosages. As the disease progresses, the therapeutic window narrows. Insufficient dosages in later disease may not bring about benefit (on). High dosages may cause choreiform dyskinesia.*

What is the "therapeutic window"?

Patients with both motor fluctuations and dyskinesia are said to have a therapeutic window. It lies above the threshold required to improve symptoms ("on threshold") and below the threshold for peak-dose dyskinesia ("dyskinesia threshold"). When patients are ON without dyskinesia they are said to be in their therapeutic window.

What happens to the therapeutic window over time?

The therapeutic window appears to become smaller over time (figure 5-2). Much of the narrowing of the therapeutic window is due to a progressive lowering of the dyskinesia threshold. Once the window is sufficiently narrowed, it may be difficult to provide much on time without dyskinesia and even optimal medication titration may do no more than provide a balance between OFF time and dyskinesia.

Which is worse, OFF time or dyskinesia?

Both OFF time and dyskinesia can be disabling. Most patients prefer dyskinesia to OFF time and most family members and physicians prefer for the patient to be off than have dyskinesia. It is important to listen to the patient and help them achieve the balance that they most prefer. Usually the goal is to maximize ON time while attempting to minimize troublesome or disabling dyskinesia. Having the patient fill out a diary divided into half-hour time periods can help the physician analyze the amount of OFF time and troublesome dyskinesia, and their relation to the timing of medication intake (figure 5-3) [9].

Are dopamine agonists associated with long term complications?

Dopamine agonists are medications that act in the brain like dopamine. Unlike levodopa, they do not need to be metabolized and they are not stored in neurons. They act at dopamine receptors in the brain to provide benefit for PD symptoms. Currently available oral dopamine agonists have relatively long half-lives of at least six hours. They therefore provide relatively continuous dopamine stimulation. Their main limitation is that they are not as efficacious as levodopa to alleviate PD symptoms especially in moderate and advanced disease. Dopamine agonists are discussed in detail in the medication chapter.

PARKINSON'S DISEASE DIARY

NAME_____   DATE_____

Instructions: For each half-hour time period place one check mark to indicate your predominant status during most of that period.
ON = Time when medication is providing benefit with regard to mobility, slowness, and stiffness.
OFF = Time when medication has worn off and is no longer providing benefit with regard to mobility, slowness, and stiffness.
Dyskinesia = Involuntary twisting, turning movements. These movements are an effect of medication and occur during ON time.
Non-troublesome dyskinesia does not interfere with function or cause meaningful discomfort. **Troublesome dyskinesia** interferes with function or causes meaningful discomfort.
Tremor is shaking back and forth and is not considered dyskinesia.

time	asleep	OFF	ON without dyskinesia	ON with non-troublesome dyskinesia	ON with troublesome dyskinesia	time	asleep	OFF	ON without dyskinesia	ON with non-troublesome dyskinesia	ON with troublesome dyskinesia
6:00 AM						6:00 PM					
:30						:30					
7:00 AM						7:00 PM					
:30						:30					
8:00 AM						8:00 PM					
:30						:30					
9:00 AM						9:00 PM					
:30						:30					
10:00 AM						10:00 PM					
:30						:30					
11:00 AM						11:00 PM					
:30						:30					
12:00 PM						12:00 AM					
:30						:30					
1:00 PM						1:00 AM					
:30						:30					
2:00 PM						2:00 AM					
:30						:30					
3:00 PM						3:00 AM					
:30						:30					
4:00 PM						4:00 AM					
:30						:30					
5:00 PM						5:00 AM					
:30						:30					

Figure 5-3. *Parkinson's disease diary.*

Motor fluctuations and dyskinesia are uncommon in patients on dopamine agonists alone (monotherapy). Agonists with long half-lives provide a relatively stable clinical response and it is unusual for a patient to experience motor fluctuations on these agents alone. However, patients with advanced disease do experience fluctuations when short-acting dopamine agonists are administered. It is also uncommon for patients to experience dyskinesia on dopamine agonist monotherapy. In contrast, patients with peak-dose dyskinesia on levodopa commonly experience a worsening of dyskinesia when an agonist is added.

Thus, it is important to differentiate emergence of dyskinesia over time, from symptomatic worsening of dyskinesia in patients who already have (or are close to having) them. Dopamine agonists alone are associated with a low incidence of the emergence of dyskinesia. In patients with dyskinesia on levodopa, the addition of a dopamine agonist commonly causes symptomatic worsening of dyskinesia.

What is the Continuous Dopaminergic Stimulation (CDS) hypothesis?

Dopamine neurons in the brain normally release dopamine in a relatively stable, or continuous, manner. In early PD, remaining dopamine neurons take up levodopa, convert it to dopamine, store it, and slowly release it. However, over time as more dopamine neurons are lost, this storage and slow release capacity is lost. Fluctuations in blood levodopa levels due to levodopa's short half-life can no longer be buffered and dopamine receptors in the brain are stimulated in an abnormal, pulsatile fashion.

The loss of intraneuronal storage and slow release capacity is expressed as a shortened duration of benefit from levodopa. Once this capacity is essentially lost, patients fluctuate in concert with levodopa fluctuations in blood.

It is thought that exposing dopamine receptors to abnormal, pulsatile stimulation causes changes that are expressed clinically as dyskinesia.

The Continuous Dopaminergic Stimulation hypothesis states that treatment strategies that provide more continuous dopaminergic stimulation cause less motor fluctuations and dyskinesia.

What is the evidence in support of the CDS hypothesis?

Support for the CDS hypothesis comes from both animal and human studies.

A large body of information comes from the MPTP monkey model of PD. Monkeys who receive MPTP, a dopamine neuron toxin, lose dopamine neurons and exhibit parkinsonian features (bradykinesia, rigidity). When treated with levodopa (which has a short half-life), they develop marked dyskinesia over several weeks. When levodopa is administered with entacapone, a COMT inhibitor that prolongs the levodopa half-life, the development of dyskinesia is reduced [10]. Further, MPTP monkeys treated with long-acting dopamine agonists develop little or no dyskinesia [11]. In contrast, short acting dopamine agonists induce dyskinesia but this can be prevented by continuous administration of the same agent.

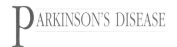

In multiple clinical trials of PD patients, initial treatment with long acting dopamine agonists (pramipexole, ropinirole, cabergoline) has caused less motor fluctuations and dyskinesia than treatment with levodopa [12,13]. These studies are discussed in detail in the medication chapter.

Is the MPTP monkey model a good model of PD?

MPTP-treated monkeys are different from Parkinson's disease patients in a number of ways. They do not have Parkinson's disease and do not experience a progressive loss of dopamine neurons over many years. MPTP causes an acute loss of dopamine neurons and when relatively high doses of MPTP are given, the extent of dopamine neuron loss is similar to that seen in advanced PD. Because of this marked loss of dopamine neurons, MPTP monkeys can develop dyskinesia over a matter of weeks, depending on the treatment.

The MPTP monkey model has thus far been highly predictive of the effects of various treatments in PD patients. It is a very useful model to determine the extent to which treatments 1) improve parkinsonian signs, and 2) cause the development of dyskiensias.

How does this information impact medical management of PD?

Younger patients are more likely than older patients to develop motor fluctuations and dyskinesia, and have a longer time horizon over which they will be treated. In contrast, older patients are somewhat less likely to develop motor fluctuations and dyskinesia and may have a shorter time horizon for treatment. In addition, older individuals are more prone to short term side-effects such as hallucinations that are more common with dopamine agonists than levodopa.

One strategy that has emerged is to initiate dopaminergic therapy in younger patients (<65?) with a dopamine agonist and to add levodopa when the dopamine agonist alone is no longer sufficient. This strategy has been demonstrated to cause less motor fluctuations and dyskinesia. When levodopa needs to be added, entacapone can be introduced at the same time in an effort to continue to reduce the development of motor fluctuations and dyskinesia. This has been suggested by MPTP monkey studies, but has not been studied in PD patients.

In older individuals (>70?), one might elect not to use dopamine agonists, but to introduce levodopa when treatment is required. As above, the use of entacapone to reduce the development of motor fluctuations and dyskinesia has been suggested by MPTP monkey studies, but not tested in PD patients.

What is freezing?

Freezing is a momentary inability to move one's feet during ambulation. Patients will describe that their feet feel stuck to the floor. Start-hesitation is freezing when a patient attempts to initiate ambulation. Freezing generally occurs late in Parkinson's disease and affects roughly one third of patients[14]. It occurs more frequently in those whose initial symptoms were gait-related. Turning or attempting to walk through a doorway may cause freezing and contribute to falls. Freezing that occurs during OFF time is improved by medication changes that reduce OFF time. Freezing during ON time is poorly responsive to medication changes. Tricks or strategies such as attempting to march rather than walk, stepping over an object, or walking over masking tape placed across a walkway may be helpful. The development of freezing appears to be related to progression of disease but its underlying pathology is not known.

CHAPTER 6

MEDICATIONS FOR THE TREATMENT OF PARKINSON'S DISEASE

When did the modern era of Parkinson's disease treatment begin?

The discovery that Parkinson's disease is associated with a striatal dopamine deficiency created new possibilities for therapeutic approaches beginning in the late 1960s. Until then, anticholinergic medications were the principal treatment and results were disappointing. Patients were subsequently found to experience dramatic benefit when placed on the dopamine precursor, levodopa[1]. Today, levodopa therapy remains the gold standard of symptomatic treatment for Parkinson's disease. However, long term therapy with levodopa is less than satisfactory as disability continues to progress and most patients develop levodopa-associated motor fluctuations and dyskinesia within a few years of treatment. Many patients ultimately develop disability due to difficulty with balance and cognition. For this reason, much research in Parkinson's disease today focuses on how to forestall disability and maintain or improve function over the long term.

What are the basic strategies used for the treatment of Parkinson's disease?

Treatment strategies are potentially divided into those that are:
a) symptomatic, b) neuroprotective, and c) restorative.

Symptomatic therapies are those that improve signs and symptoms without affecting the underlying disease state. Degeneration of the substantia nigra in Parkinson's disease causes a striatal dopamine deficiency. Administration of levodopa increases dopamine concentration in the striatum. Levodopa is administered in combination with a peripheral decarboxylase inhibitor (PDI) to minimize nausea.

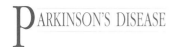

Catechol-O-methyltransferase (COMT) inhibitors further inhibit levodopa's peripheral metabolism, thereby enhancing central bioavailability. Selegiline increases dopamine activity in the brain by inhibiting its metabolism. Dopamine agonists provide symptomatic benefit by directly stimulating post-synaptic striatal dopamine receptors. Other medications used in the treatment of Parkinson's disease include amantadine, which augments dopamine release and anticholinergics such as trihexyphenidyl and benztropine, which block striatal cholinergic function. Each of these medications is discussed in greater detail below.

Neuroprotective therapies are those that slow neuronal degeneration, thereby delaying disease progression. Currently, there are no proven neuroprotective therapies available for Parkinson's disease. New medications are now being evaluated for their ability to slow disease progression.

Restorative therapies are those that aim to replace lost neurons. One approach to replacing lost neurons is the transplantation of cells. Transplanted cells have been demonstrated to survive, restore neuronal connections, and increase dopamine concentration. However, transplantation has not been demonstrated to provide benefit for patients. Stem cells, genetically engineered cells, and cells from other parts of the human body are being developed for transplantation and will be evaluated for possible restorative effects.

What is levodopa?

Levodopa is the chemical precursor of dopamine. The dopamine depletor reserpine was found to produce parkinsonian symptoms in rats in the late 1950s [2]. In addition, post-mortem examinations of Parkinson's disease patients revealed decreased dopamine concentration in the striatum, correlating with the loss of nigro-striatal neurons in the substantia nigra [3]. As dopamine does not cross the blood-brain barrier, its precursor, levodopa, was tested as dopamine replacement therapy. Levodopa was shown to dramatically improve parkinsonian symptoms [4].

The main difficulty with early levodopa therapy was the high incidence of nausea and vomiting. Concomitant administration of peripheral decarboxylase inhibitors was found to improve the clinical utility of levodopa by reducing its peripheral breakdown [5]. Decreased peripheral dopamine production reduced the incidence of nausea and vomiting and allowed more levodopa to cross the blood-brain barrier. The decarboxylase inhibitors carbidopa and benserazide are most commonly combined with levodopa for this purpose.

What are the pharmacokinetics of levodopa?

Levodopa, or l-dihydroxyphenylalanine, is a large neutral amino acid. After oral ingestion, it is absorbed in the proximal small intestine by a saturable, carrier-mediated transport system. Absorption can be delayed by meals [6] and increased gastric acidity [7]. Absorbed levodopa is not bound to plasma protein and its half-life is approximately one hour [8]. To exert an anti-parkinsonian effect, levodopa must cross the blood-brain barrier by way of the large neutral amino acid carrier transport system.

What is levodopa/carbidopa?

Levodopa/carbidopa (Sinemet®) is a combination of carbidopa, a peripheral decarboxylase inhibitor, and levodopa. Carbidopa lessens the extracerebral decarboxylation of levodopa, thereby decreasing the incidence of nausea and increasing the central availability of levodopa. The addition of carbidopa reduces the amount of levodopa needed by about 75% [9]. Approximately 75 to 100 mg of carbidopa are required to saturate peripheral decarboxylase [5]. Nonetheless, some patients require carbidopa in doses up to 200 mg per day to reduce or eliminate nausea. The half-life of levodopa when administered with carbidopa is approximately 90 minutes [9].

Standard levodopa/carbidopa can be taken with or without meals. When taken with or shortly after a meal, its absorption is mildly decreased and delayed. Patients with early PD usually find that the levodopa benefit lasts from dose to dose (stable response) and these individuals will usually not notice any difference in benefit taking levodopa/carbidopa with or without a meal. If such a patient experiences nausea in association with levodopa/carbidopa intake, taking the medication just after a meal commonly helps reduce the nausea.

In contrast, patients with moderate or advanced disease who find that benefit from levodopa wears off prior to the next dose taking effect, will often find that the benefit is less and won't last as long if they take it with a meal. Therefore, levodopa/carbidopa is usually administered one half hour or more before, or one hour or more after meals to achieve the most consistent absorption and greatest clinical benefit.

Although levodopa competes with other large, neutral amino acids (proteins) for transport across the blood-brain barrier, only patients with bothersome motor fluctuations on levodopa/carbidopa need to consider a low protein or protein redistributed diet.

Are generic forms of levodopa/carbidopa available and do they have the same effect?

Generic forms of Sinemet are available in the United States. Generics may contain slightly less or slightly more levodopa. Most patients do not notice a difference between generic and brand formulations, however, 20-30% of patients, especially those with motor fluctuations may notice worsening of symptoms when changing to a generic formulation [10,11].

What is levodopa/benserazide?

Levodopa/benserazide (Madopar®) is a combination of benserazide, a peripheral decarboxylase inhibitor, and levodopa. It is used similarly to levodopa/carbidopa. This preparation is available outside the United States.

How do I initiate standard levodopa/carbidopa?

A commonly used initial target dose is carbidopa/levodopa 25/100 three times a day (TID), starting with half of a 25/100 tablet each day for the first week and increasing by a half tablet per day each week until the target dose is reached. The final dose must be tailored to the individual patient. If there is a need to improve symptoms more quickly, the dose can potentially be increased by half of a 25/100 tablet every 2-3 days. The "start low" and "go slow" regimen helps avoid side-effects such as nausea.

What are the side-effects of levodopa/carbidopa and levodopa/benserazide?

The most common side effect of levodopa/carbidopa and levodopa/benserazide is nausea. This is due to stimulation of the vomiting center in the medulla by dopamine formed in the bloodstream. If a patient has difficulty initiating the medication due to nausea, they should try taking it with a carbohydrate snack or immediately following a meal. Additional carbidopa (Lodosyn®) may be prescribed. These steps will allow the vast majority of patients to tolerate these medications without much difficulty. Where available, the use of a peripherally acting dopamine blocking drug, such as domperidone (Motilium®) is very helpful to alleviate refractory nausea.

Other potential side-effects include orthostatic hypotension (lightheadedness), confusion, hallucinations, delusions, and sleepiness. Orthostatic hypotension can usually be countered with medications such as fludrocortisone (Florinef®) or midodrine (Proamatine®)[12]. Cognitive side-effects typically occur later in the disease in patients who have developed underlying dementia. Confusion may occasionally improve with a decrease in levodopa dose. Hallucinations and delusions can be treated with atypical neuroleptics with minimal parkinsonian side-effects (see below).

What is levodopa/carbidopa Extended Release (ER)?

Levodopa/carbidopa ER (Sinemet CR®) is a controlled-release preparation. It is more slowly absorbed and provides more sustained serum levels than standard levodopa/carbidopa[13]. It is best absorbed when taken with food and levodopa bioavailability is about 75-80% that of standard levodopa/carbidopa[14]. One potential drawback is that it takes about a half an hour longer to begin to exert its effect. This has no noticeable effect in early PD, but patients with more advanced PD may notice a delayed kick in.

The initial target dose is carbidopa/levodopa ER 25/100 TID or 50/200 BID, usually starting with 100 mg levodopa per day and slowly increasing over a period of a few weeks. To convert a patient from standard levodopa/carbidopa to levodopa/carbidopa ER, the daily dosage is increased by approximately 20-25% while the number of daily doses is decreased by 30-50%[15,16].

Patients with moderate or advanced disease who experience a delayed kick in of effect on levodopa/carbidopa ER often need a small amount of standard levodopa/carbidopa as part of the first morning dose to act as a "booster" and bring on symptomatic benefit more quickly. This is often accomplished by adding one carbidopa/levodopa 25/100 tablet to the first ER dose of the day. Patients on standard carbidopa/levodopa who need a bedtime dose often use the ER formulation for that dose so that benefit into the night will be more prolonged.

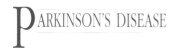

What are the side-effects of levodopa/carbidopa ER?

Side-effects of levodopa/carbidopa ER are similar to those of standard levodopa/carbidopa. However, because levodopa/carbidopa ER persists longer in the blood, acute transient side-effects may also persist longer with levodopa/carbidopa ER. For example, a patient who experiences nausea or lightheadedness for a half-hour after taking standard levodopa/carbidopa may have those side-effects for an hour after taking levodopa/carbidopa ER. However, when given the same mg strength ER vs. standard tablets, some patients will find that such symptoms are diminished on the ER formulation because of its lower bioavailability.

What is levodopa/carbidopa/entacapone?

Levodopa/carbidopa/entacapone (Stalevo®) is a combination of standard levodopa/carbidopa plus entacapone. Entacapone (Comtan®, Comtess®), also available as a separate product, is a catechol-O-methyltransferase (COMT) inhibitor. COMT is one of the main enzymes responsible for levodopa's metabolism and clearance from the blood. The addition of entacapone to standard levodopa/carbidopa prolongs the levodopa half-life to approximately 2.25 hours[9]. This provides more sustained levels of levodopa in the blood.

In moderate and advanced patients with motor fluctuations, the addition of entacapone to levodopa/carbidopa and similarly, switching from levodopa/carbidopa to levodopa/carbidopa/entacapone reduces OFF time and helps smooth the clinical response. Levodopa/carbidopa/entacapone provides as quick an onset of action as standard levodopa/carbidopa but lasts longer. Entacapone is discussed in more detail later in this chapter.

There is also interest in the use of levodopa/carbidopa/entacapone as initial levodopa therapy. In the MPTP monkey model of PD, administration of entacapone with levodopa/carbidopa on a QID schedule caused significantly less dyskinesia than levodopa/carbidopa administered QID without entacapone or the same daily dose of levodopa/carbidopa divided BID with or without entacapone[17]. These findings are consistent with the Continuous Dopaminergic Stimulation hypothesis.

Levodopa/carbidopa/entacapone, when used as initial levodopa therapy is usually initiated at a dose of one 50/12.5/200 mg tablet (50 mg levodopa) or one 100/25/200 mg tablet (100 mg levodopa) per day and increased by one tablet a day each week to a TID or QID schedule. Side-effects are similar to other levodopa preparations.

When I begin levodopa should I use standard levodopa/carbidopa, levodopa/carbidopa ER, or levodopa/carbidopa/entacapone?

Standard levodopa/carbidopa, levodopa/carbidopa ER, and levodopa/carbidopa/entacapone are equally effective in improving motor symptoms when levodopa is first required. Generic formulations of standard and ER levodopa/carbidopa are available and are less expensive than the brand formulations. Patients find the levodopa/carbidopa ER or levodopa/carbidopa/entacapone more convenient because fewer daily doses may be required. There is interest as to whether more continuous dopamine receptor stimulation as afforded by levodopa/carbidopa ER or levodopa/carbidopa/entacapone can forestall the development of long term complications including motor fluctuations and dyskinesia. A five-year study comparing standard and ER levodopa/carbidopa found no difference in the incidence of fluctuations and dyskinesia [17b]. However, levodopa/carbidopa ER was administered on a BID schedule in that study and that may be too infrequent to provide sufficiently continuous stimulation. Levodopa/carbidopa/entacapone administered on a QID schedule to MPTP monkeys caused less motor fluctuations and dyskinesia the levodopa/carbidopa QID or the same daily levodopa/carbidopa dose administered BID with or without entacapone [17].

Once patients develop troublesome motor fluctuations and dyskinesia, levodopa/carbidopa ER becomes more problematic because of variability in its absorption. Standard levodopa formulations (levodopa/carbidopa and levodopa/carbidopa/entacapone) provide a more consistent response.

What is levodopa/benserazide HBS?

Levodopa/benserazide hydrodynamically balanced system (Madopar HBS®) is a controlled-release levodopa preparation available outside the U.S. containing hydrocolloids, fats, and the decarboxylase inhibitor benserazide. Levodopa/benserazide HBS "floats" on stomach contents for five to twelve hours allowing levodopa to be slowly absorbed. Compared to standard levodopa/benserazide, levodopa bioavailability is about 60%, so a switch usually necessitates a dosage increase [18]. As with other controlled-release preparations, it is often supplemented with a small dose of the standard formulation to provide an early morning "kick".

What symptoms of Parkinson's disease are best alleviated by levodopa therapy?

Levodopa therapy is the cornerstone of symptomatic treatment. It is most effective in relieving bradykinesia and rigidity, while its effect on tremor is highly variable [19]. Symptoms such as balance impairment and dementia are not alleviated by levodopa. Depression, freezing, autonomic nervous system dysfunction, and pain are sometimes helped by levodopa.

When assessing the benefit of levodopa, one should evaluate motor function, specifically bradykinesia and rigidity. Symptomatic improvement may or may not occur if a patient only has tremor. In addition, improvement may be difficult to detect if symptoms are minimal. Improvement with levodopa therapy is usually apparent with more advanced disease as motor dysfunction, bradykinesia, and rigidity become more obvious.

What are COMT inhibitors?

Catechol-O-methyltransferase (COMT) is one of the main enzymes responsible for the metabolism of levodopa, dopamine, other catecholamines (adrenaline and noradrenaline), and their metabolites. COMT catalyzes the transfer of a methyl group from S-adenosyl-L-methionine (SAM) to the hydroxyl group of catecholamines (figure 6-1) [53].

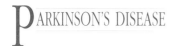

Figure 6-1. *Methylation of catechol substrate by COMT.*
SAM = S-adenosyl-L-methionine; SAH = S-adenosyl-L-homocysteine; R = side chain.

COMT is widely distributed throughout the body [54,55] including central nervous system neurons and glia, but not nigrostriatal dopamine neurons [56].

Levodopa is metabolized by several different enzymes (figure 6-2), with dopa decarboxylase and COMT being most important. When levodopa is administered with a peripheral dopa decarboxylase inhibitor such as carbidopa or benserazide, COMT metabolism of levodopa predominates. COMT metabolizes levodopa to 3-O-methyldopa (3-OMD). 3-OMD has the potential to decrease levodopa absorption and efficacy [57,58], although at the concentrations present in PD patients, this does not appear to be an

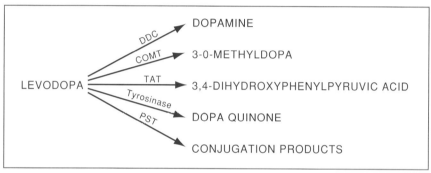

Figure 6-2. *The metabolism of levodopa.*
DDC = dopa decarboxylase; COMT = catechol-O-methyltransferase;
TAT = tyrosine aminotransferase; PST = phenol sulphotransferase.

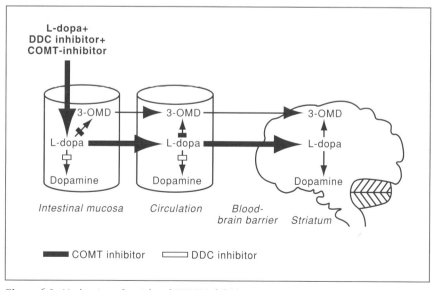

Figure 6-3. *Mechanism of peripheral COMT inhibition.*

important consideration. Peripherally acting COMT inhibitors block COMT in the gut and periphery. By decreasing levodopa metabolism, they make more levodopa available for transport across the blood-brain barrier over a longer time and also reduce 3-OMD production (figure 6-3)[59]. When COMT inhibitors are added to levodopa therapy, striatal dopamine concentrations increase[59]. Central COMT inhibition might further increase striatal dopamine concentration by inhibiting the metabolism of dopamine to homovanillic acid (HVA)[59].

What is entacapone?

Entacapone (Comtan®,Comtess®) is a reversible peripheral COMT inhibitor (figure 6-4)[60]. Its half-life is approximately one half hour (0.4-0.7 hrs)[61]. Entacapone is usually administered at a dose of 200 mg with each levodopa dose, up to a maximum of eight times a day (1600 mg). Entacapone reduces the peripheral metabolism of levodopa to 3-OMD[61], prolongs the levodopa half-life from 1.3 to 2.4 hours and increases levodopa availability (area under the curve) by approximately 35%[62].

Side-effects are mostly those related to increased dopaminergic stimulation. Dyskinesia may emerge or worsen when entacapone is added, and some

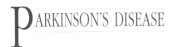

Figure 6-4. *The structures of entacapone and tolcapone.*

patients may require a reduction in levodopa dose, usually on the order of 10-25%. Those patients likely to require a reduction in levodopa dose are those who have moderate or severe dyskinesia on levodopa alone and to a lesser extent, those on more than 600-800 mg levodopa/day. Other dopaminergic side-effects include nausea and hallucinations. These side-effects can usually be reduced or eliminated by decreasing the levodopa dose. Approximately 10% of patients experience diarrhea and 2% discontinue entacapone because of this side effect. Onset of diarrhea typically occurs within 4-12 weeks but may be earlier or later. The mechanism of this side effect is unknown. Patients should be informed that they might notice a brownish orange discoloration of the urine or sweat that is not clinically relevant.

There is no known hepatotoxicity associated with entacapone and there is no requirement for liver function test monitoring. In clinical trials, elevations of liver function tests were no more common in entacapone-treated patients than placebo-treated patients.

Entacapone is effective in reducing OFF time, improving motor function, and allowing levodopa dose reductions in patients with motor fluctuations on levodopa. The Parkinson Study Group (PSG) conducted a multicenter, double-blind, placebo-controlled trial of entacapone in 205 fluctuating PD patients over a 24-week period [63]. This trial is known as SEESAW (Safety and Efficacy of Entacapone Study Assessing Wearing Off). Patients were randomized to receive either entacapone 200 mg or placebo with each levodopa dose. OFF time was reduced by 17.6% in entacapone-treated patients compared to 4.5% in placebo-treated patients (p<0.01). The total daily levodopa dose was decreased by 11.6% in the entacapone group compared to an increase of 2.5% in the placebo group (p<0.001). UPDRS ADL, motor, and total scores all improved significantly.

A similar study design was used in the NOMECOMT (Nordic Multicenter Entacapone COMT) trial [64]. In entacapone-treated patients, mean OFF time decreased by 22% (p < 0.001) and mean ON time increased by more than 13% (p < 0.01). UPDRS scores improved significantly and daily levodopa dose and intake frequency were significantly reduced.

In an open-label extension of the NOMECOMT study, called NOMESAFE, 92% of patients maintained benefit regarding OFF time through three years.

At three years when entacapone was withdrawn, symptoms worsened, demonstrating that entacapone was still providing benefit [64b].

In a multi-center double-blind, placebo-controlled study, entacapone was evaluated as an adjunct to levodopa in 750 patients who were experiencing a stable motor response (i.e. no motor fluctuations). Although entacapone did not improve motor function in these patients, it was associated with a significant improvement in quality of life. There were no differences between entacapone and placebo in serious adverse effects [65].

What is tolcapone?

Tolcapone (Tasmar®) is a reversible COMT inhibitor (figure 6-4). It has the capacity to induce fatal hepatic failure and strict liver function test monitoring is required. Because of this risk, its use is reserved for patients with motor fluctuations on levodopa who do not respond to or who could not tolerate other adjunctive therapies. Animal studies indicate that tolcapone exerts central as well as peripheral COMT inhibition [59]. It is rapidly absorbed and has a half-life of approximately two hours [66]. It is introduced at a dose of 100 mg TID and this is the usual maintenance dose. The dose can be increased to 200 mg TID in selected patients in whom the additional benefit is felt to outweigh the additional risk.

Other side-effects are mostly those related to increased dopaminergic stimulation [67]. Patients with levodopa-induced dyskinesia often have an initial rapid increase in dyskinesia necessitating a 25-50% reduction in levodopa dose. Alternatively, the levodopa dose can be reduced by 25-50% at the time tolcapone is initiated and then titrated further as appropriate. Additional dopaminergic side-effects include nausea and hallucinations. These side-effects can usually be reduced or eliminated by decreasing the levodopa dose. Approximately 10% of patients experience diarrhea and 3% discontinue tolcapone because of this side effect. Onset of diarrhea is usually delayed for four to twelve weeks after initiation of therapy but uncommon after six months [67].

Tolcapone improves motor function and allows levodopa dose reductions in patients on levodopa therapy with either motor fluctuations or a stable response. Two studies evaluated the efficacy of adding tolcapone to levodopa therapy in patients experiencing motor fluctuations [68,69]. OFF time was reduced by two hours per day in patients taking 100 mg TID and 2.5 hours per day in patients taking 200 mg TID [69].

In a double-blind, placebo-controlled study evaluating tolcapone in 298 patients on levodopa without motor fluctuations, tolcapone produced significant reductions in activities of daily living and motor function at both 100 mg TID and 200 mg TID dosing. These improvements were maintained up to 12 months [67]. However, tolcapone is not indicated for use in patients without motor fluctuations because the benefit does not appear to justify the risk.

Does tolcapone cause liver damage?

In clinical trials, hepatic enzymes alanine aminotransferase (ALT) and aspartate aminotransferase (AST), were elevated to more than three times the upper limits of normal in approximately 1% and 3% of patients treated with tolcapone 100 mg TID and 200 mg TID, respectively. Increases to more than eight times the upper limits of normal occurred in 0.3% and 0.7% of patients. Women were more likely than men to experience an increase in hepatic enzymes (approximately 5% versus 2%). Elevations usually occurred within six weeks to six months of starting treatment. When tolcapone was discontinued, enzymes generally returned to normal within two to three weeks, but in some cases took as long as one to two months. None of the patients in clinical trials developed clinical sequelae of liver injury.

Tolcapone became available for clinical use in August of 1997 in Europe, and in February, 1998 in the U.S. By October, 1998, three cases of fatal hepatic failure were identified from approximately sixty thousand patients on tolcapone, providing approximately forty thousand patient-years of worldwide use [70]. This incidence was approximately 10-100 times higher than the background incidence of fatal hepatic failure in the general population. All three patients were women in their seventies who were placed on tolcapone but did not undergo liver function monitoring. Time from initiation of tolcapone to clinical illness ranged form eight to twelve weeks. Recognition of the potential for life-threatening hepatocellular injury prompted the withdrawal of tolcapone in Europe, and in the U.S. the FDA revised the labeling. This labeling change emphasized the need for rigorous liver function enzyme monitoring.

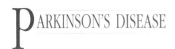

The risks of tolcapone use should be reviewed with the patient and the patient should provide written informed consent. ALT/AST levels should be obtained at baseline, every two weeks for the first year of therapy, every four weeks for the next six months, and then every eight weeks for the duration of administration. Tolcapone should be discontinued if ALT/AST exceeds the upper limit of normal. If meaningful clinical benefit is not observed within three weeks, tolcapone should be discontinued.

What are dopamine agonists?

Dopamine agonists directly stimulate post-synaptic dopamine receptors and unlike levodopa they do not require enzymatic conversion[20]. They provide symptomatic benefit as monotherapy in early disease and as adjuncts to levodopa in later disease.

What are the side-effects of dopamine agonists?

Dopamine agonists can cause nausea, vomiting, and orthostatic hypotension by stimulating peripheral dopamine receptors. They may also cause central dopaminergic side-effects such as nightmares, hallucinations, or psychiatric symptoms. Cognitive side-effects are dose related but nausea and orthostatic hypotension can occur even with small initial doses. Other possible side-effects include leg edema and constipation[21].

Should dopamine agonists be given with or without food?

Meals have little effect on the extent of absorption of dopamine agonists and they can be taken with or without food. Patients with nausea should take their medication after a meal. For patients on combination therapy with levodopa, the dopamine agonist is usually scheduled to be taken with levodopa as a matter of convenience.

What is bromocriptine?

Bromocriptine (Parlodel®) is an ergot alkaloid dopamine receptor agonist (figure 6-5). It is a strong D2 receptor agonist and a weak D1 receptor antagonist (6-6). It stimulates both pre- and post-synaptic receptors, and its half-life is approximately seven hours[9]. It can be initiated at a dose of one half of a 2.5 mg tablet per day, and increased every third day by 2.5 mg to a daily dose in the range of 10-40 mg[21]. A TID dosing schedule is typically used. Potential side-effects include nausea, vomiting, orthostatic

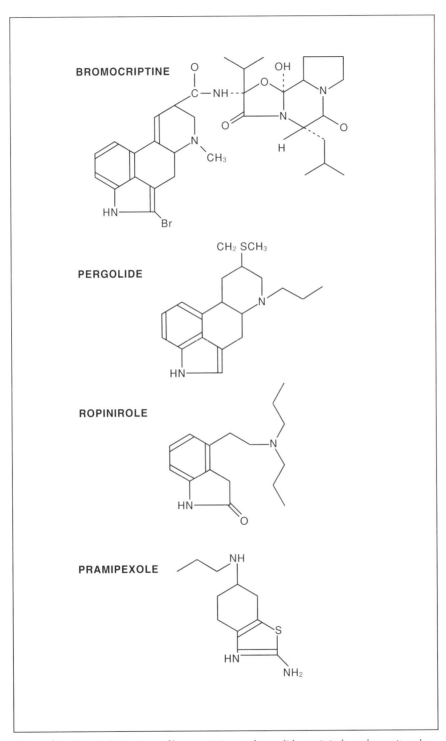

Figure 6-5. *Chemical structures of bromocriptine and pergolide, ropinirole and pramipexole.*

			Receptor Binding			
	D_2	D_3	D_1	$5HT_{1/2}$	α_1	α_2
Bromocriptine[1]	++	+	+	++	++	++
Pergolide[2]	++	++	++	++	+	++
Ropinirole	++	+++	-	-	-	-
Pramipexole	++	+++	-	-	-	-
[1] Bromocriptine is a D_1 Antagonist [2] Pergolide is a D_1 Agonist						

Figure 6-6. *Receptor binding of bromocriptine, pergolide, ropinirole and pramipexole.*

hypotension, confusion, hallucinations, anorexia, and erythromelalgia, a painful, reddish discoloration of the skin. Retroperitoneal fibrosis has been reported in a few patients who received long term therapy at high dosages.

What is pergolide?

Pergolide (Permax®) is a semisynthetic, clavine ergot derivative dopamine agonist (figure 6-5). In contrast to bromocriptine, it is a strong D2 receptor agonist and a weak D1 receptor agonist (figure 6-6). Peak plasma levels are achieved in one to two hours, and its half-life is approximately 20-27 hours[9]. The starting dose is 0.05 mg tablet per day, with an initial target dose of 0.25 mg TID achieved over 4-6 weeks. The usual maximum recommended dose is 4-5 mg per day in divided doses. Potential side-effects include nausea, vomiting, orthostatic hypotension, cognitive dysfunction, increased liver enzymes, erythromelalgia, and peripheral edema[22]. A recent report noted valvular heart disease in three patients taking pergolide[23]. This potential side effect appears to be rare, but it seems prudent to obtain an echocardiogram of the heart intermittently in patients chronically treated with pergolide.

Pergolide was compared to placebo as an adjunct to levodopa in patients with motor fluctuations[21]. Pergolide permitted a mean levodopa dose reduction of 24.7% compared with 4.9% in the placebo group (p < .001). Motor function improved by 35% in pergolide-treated patients compared with 17% in placebo-treated patients (p < .001) and OFF time decreased by 32% compared with 4% (p < .001). Although new onset or worsening of dyskinesia was observed in 62% of the pergolide group compared to 25% of the placebo group, dyskinesia was generally controlled by a reduction of levodopa dose such that there was no difference in dyskinesia disability by the end of the study.

What is ropinirole?

Ropinirole (Requip®) is a highly selective D2 agonist with little affinity for
D1, 5HT, muscarinic, or adrenergic receptors (figure 6-6). It is a non-ergoline
dopamine agonist and has a half-life of approximately six hours (figure 6-5).
Maximal plasma concentration is reached approximately 1.5 hours after
administration in fasted patients and approximately four hours when taken
with meals [25]. The starting dose is 0.25 mg TID, with an initial target dose of
3 mg TID achieved over 8 weeks. Further escalation should be undertaken as
clinically necessary with a recommended maximum dose of 24 mg per day.
Side-effects are similar to other dopamine agonists and include nausea,
somnolence, insomnia, dizziness, dyspepsia, and headache [21].

Ropinirole is effective both as early monotherapy and as an adjunct to
treatment with levodopa. There have been a number of studies
demonstrating the safety and efficacy of ropinirole in the treatment of
Parkinson's disease. One study compared ropinirole to placebo as add-on
therapy in patients not optimally controlled on levodopa. At six months,
27.7% of ropinirole-treated patients had at least a 20% reduction in levodopa
dose and at least a 20% reduction in OFF time compared with 11% in the
placebo group (odds ratio = 4.4; 95% confidence interval, 1.53 to 12.66) [26].
Mean reduction of levodopa dose in the ropinirole group was 19.4%.

In a study of ropinirole as monotherapy in early stage patients, motor
function was improved by 24% at six months in ropinirole-treated patients
compared with a 3% worsening in placebo-treated patients ($p < .001$)[27].
Significantly fewer ropinirole-treated patients required levodopa compared
with placebo-treated patients (11% vs. 29%, $p < 0.001$). In a six-month study
comparing ropinirole with levodopa in early stage patients, a similar
percentage of patients in each group experienced greater than 30%
improvement (48% vs. 58%), although levodopa-treated patients experienced
significantly greater improvement overall (32% vs. 44%) [28].

Ropinirole has been demonstrated to reduce the incidence of dyskinesia
when used in early PD [29]. In a 5-year study, 268 de-novo PD patients were
randomized to receive levodopa or ropinirole to which levodopa could be
added if necessary. At the completion of the study, patients in both groups
had experienced benefit in parkinsonian symptoms, however, the benefit was
significantly greater for those in the levodopa compared to the ropinirole
group ($p < 0.008$). On the other hand, dyskinesia had developed in only 20%

of patients in the ropinirole group compared to 45% in the levodopa group (p < 0.001). Patients in the ropinirole group also developed significantly less disabling dyskinesia. Adverse effects such as hallucinations, somnolence and peripheral edema were more common in the ropinirole group. This study suggests that the strategy of starting symptomatic therapy with ropinirole and then adding levodopa later when necessary leads to less dyskinesia [29].

Does ropinirole slow the progression of PD?

One way to assess PD progression is by neuroimaging. 18F-dopa PET scans evaluate the amount of dopa that is taken up by remaining dopamine neurons and serves as an index of the number of remaining dopamine neurons. β-CIT SPECT scans evaluate the amount of β-CIT that binds to dopamine reuptake sites on dopamine neuron terminals and also serves as an index of the number of remaining dopamine neurons.

The REAL-PET [30] study was a two-year, double-blind, multi-national study in which 186 PD patients with no previous dopaminergic treatment participated. Patients were randomized to treatment with either levodopa or ropinirole to which open label levodopa could be added if necessary. The primary endpoint was the change in putamen 18F-dopa uptake on positron emission tomography (PET). There were 68 (74%) patients who completed the ropinirole arm and 69 (76%) who completed the levodopa arm. The change in 18F-dopa uptake at the end of the study compared to baseline was -13% for the ropinirole arm and -20% for the levodopa arm. This is a relative difference of 35%, suggesting a slower disease progression with ropinirole compared to levodopa. However, direct pharmacologic effects of these medications, or compensatory mechanisms cannot be excluded as possible alternative explanations for these results. Three percent of patients on ropinirole versus 27% on levodopa developed dyskinesia, however, patients on levodopa had significantly greater motor improvement.

What is pramipexole?

Pramipexole (Mirapex®) is a non-ergot D2/D3 agonist (figure 6-6). It is a synthetic amino-benzathiazol derivative that binds to D3 receptors with 7-fold greater affinity than to D2 or D4 receptors and has little affinity for D1, 5HT, muscarinic, or adrenergic receptors [31]. Pramipexole is introduced at a dose of 0.125 mg TID for one week and escalated over three weeks to an initial target dose of 0.5 mg TID. The usual recommended maximum dose is 4.5 mg/day. Side-effects are similar to other dopamine agonists and include somnolence, nausea, constipation, insomnia, and hallucinations [32,33].

Pramipexole is effective both as early monotherapy and as an adjunct to treatment with levodopa. In a comparison of pramipexole to placebo as monotherapy in early disease, pramipexole significantly improved motor function and activities of daily living [32]. In a six-month trial comparing pramipexole to placebo as add-on therapy in patients with motor fluctuations on levodopa, "off" time was reduced by 17% in pramipexole-treated patients compared with 8% in placebo-treated patients (p < .01) [33]. Levodopa was reduced by 25% in the pramipexole group compared with 6% in the placebo group (p < .01). An open-label extension found that pramipexole demonstrated continued efficacy as an adjunct to levodopa for up to three years. After three years there was a gradual return to baseline motor disability consistent with disease progression. Common side-effects in this long term study included dyskinesia, dizziness, insomnia and hallucinations [34].

Pramipexole has been demonstrated to reduce the incidence of dyskinesia and motor fluctuations when used in early PD [35]. The CALM-PD study was a two year study in which 301 patients with early PD who required dopaminergic therapy were randomized to receive either pramipexole or levodopa to which levodopa could be added if necessary. At the conclusion of the study, patients assigned to levodopa had greater improvement in motor function compared to pramipexole. However, 28% of patients on pramipexole developed wearing off, dyskinesia or on-off motor fluctuations compared to 51% on levodopa. This result is consistent with the Continuous Dopaminergic Stimulation hypothesis. Somnolence, hallucinations and peripheral edema were were more common in the pramipexole group than the levodopa group.

Does pramipexole slow the progression of PD?

The ability of pramipexole to slow disease progression was evaluated using β-CIT SPECT scanning as an index of remaining dopamine neurons in the CALM-PD-CIT study [36]. This study included a subset of patients from the CALM-PD study. Eighty-two patients received a single photon computed emission tomography (SPECT) scan at baseline and at regular intervals during the study. The primary outcome measure was the change from baseline in striatal [123I] β-CIT uptake, a marker of dopamine neuron degeneration, at

46 months. The percent loss in striatal β-CIT uptake was significantly reduced in the pramipexole group compared to the levodopa group (~40%), suggesting slower disease progression in the pramipexole group compared to the levodopa group. However, direct pharmacologic effects of these medications, or compensatory mechanisms cannot be excluded as possible alternative explanations for these results.

What is cabergoline?

Cabergoline (Cabaser®) is a long-acting ergot derivative agonist with a high affinity for D2 receptors[37]. Its biological half-life is approximately sixty-five hours[38] and it is usually administered as a once a day dose. Cabergoline can be introduced at a dose of 0.05 mg and titrated to a usual maximum of 5 mg once daily. Side-effects are similar to other agonists and include dizziness, hypersomnolence, headache, nausea, and orthostatic hypotension[39].

In a six-month study comparing cabergoline to placebo as adjunctive therapy to levodopa for patients with motor fluctuations, cabergoline allowed an 18% reduction in levodopa dose compared with 3% in placebo-treated patients (p < .001)[40]. Motor function improved 16% in the cabergoline group compared with 6% in the control group (p = .031). ON time was significantly increased (p = .02) and associated with a corresponding decrease in OFF time and ON time with dyskinesia.

Are there other dopamine agonists?

Lisuride is a hydrophilic semisynthetic ergot alkaloid dopamine agonist. It stimulates D2 and 5-HT (serotonin) receptors[41]. When given orally its half-life is one and a half to two hours. It is water-soluble and can also be administered subcutaneously or by continuous intravenous infusion to help ameliorate severe motor fluctuations[42,43].

Apomorphine is a D2 and D1 receptor agonist. It is highly lipophilic and usually administered subcutaneously. Onset of action is within five to fifteen minutes and its effect lasts 90 to 120 minutes[44]. Because of its rapid onset of action, it can be used as a rescue agent for refractory off periods. Anti-emetics such as domperidone are helpful to reduce associated nausea and vomiting[45,46].

What are the advantages of using dopamine agonists?

There are two main concerns regarding chronic levodopa therapy:
1) dopamine's oxidative metabolism may lead to free radical formation and cause or accelerate neuronal degeneration, and 2) rapidly fluctuating levels of levodopa-derived dopamine may sensitize dopamine receptors and lead to dyskinesia. Unlike levodopa, dopamine agonists directly stimulate post-synaptic dopamine receptors. They do not undergo oxidative metabolism and there is no evidence that they might accelerate the disease process.

Bromocriptine, pergolide, ropinirole, pramipexole, and cabergoline all have significantly longer half-lives than levodopa and do not expose receptors to rapidly fluctuating levels of stimulation. Several prospective studies have found that initial treatment with a dopamine agonist followed by the addition of levodopa when necessary is associated with a lower prevalence of dyskinesia [29,35,47,48].

The main limitation of dopamine agonist monotherapy is that symptoms are adequately controlled for a period of only one to five years. Rinne found that after three years of bromocriptine monotherapy only 28%, and after five years only 7%, of patients were still adequately maintained on monotherapy alone [49]. In the ropinirole five-year study, 54% of ropinirole-assigned patients remaining in the study at three years and 34% at five years were still on monotherapy [29]. After a few years, most patients require the addition of levodopa to sustain good benefit.

In moderate and advanced disease, dopamine agonists provide benefit for patients with motor fluctuations on levodopa therapy. When an agonist is added, OFF time is reduced, motor function is improved and levodopa doses may be reduced. Only rarely can a patient with fluctuations and dyskinesia on levodopa be adequately managed with dopamine agonists alone.

How do I switch from one dopamine agonist to another?

One can switch directly from one agonist to another by substituting potency equivalent doses. Alternatively, a patient can be tapered off one agonist before introducing another at a low dose and escalating upward. The mg potency ratio of the various agonists is: 10 mg bromocriptine = 1 mg of pergolide = 1 mg of pramipexole = 1 mg of cabergoline = 3 mg of ropinirole.

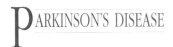

Can I abruptly stop dopaminergic medications?

Dopaminergic medications (levodopa preparations and dopamine agonists) should generally not be abruptly discontinued. Although many patients will tolerate abrupt withdrawal without difficulty, there is the possibility that a rare patient may experience neuroleptic malignant syndrome, a potentially fatal condition.

Is excessive daytime sleepiness related to dopamine agonist use?

Excessive daytime sleepiness (EDS) is a concern in PD patients as it may cause unintended episodes of sleep and lead to traffic accidents or other injuries. A complete sleep history including the Epworth Sleepiness Scale can be helpful in identifying persons at risk for EDS. Although EDS was initially attributed to pramipexole and ropinirole use [50], it is now clear that any dopaminergic medication can cause sleepiness, and other factors may also be involved.

In a study of 638 highly functional PD patients without dementia in which 420 were active drivers, EDS was reported in 51% of patients and 51% of active drivers. There were no differences in the sleepiness scores or the risk of falling asleep while driving with regard to the particular dopamine agonist used [51]. In a study of 303 PD patients, the factors most highly predictive of EDS were longer disease duration, more advanced disease,

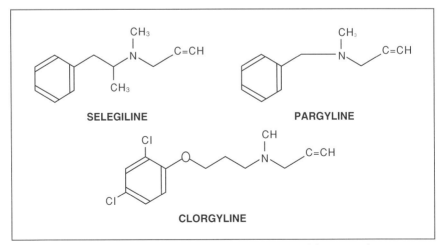

Figure 6-7. *Chemical structures of selegiline, a selective MAO-B inhibitor; pargyline, a non-selective MAO inhibitor; and clorgyline, a selective MAO-A inhibitor.*

male gender and use of any dopamine agonist[52]. However, falling asleep while driving was best predicted by older age, use of levodopa and use of any dopamine agonist[52].

It seems prudent that patients who doze off while driving or who fall asleep during activities such as working, eating or holding a conversation should not drive. If a particular medication can be identified that might be causing sleepiness consideration can be given to reducing or discontinuing it. It should also be recalled that PD patients do experience sleep disorders such as sleep apnea, and a polysomnogram can help identify these conditions.

What is selegiline?

Selegiline is a relatively selective, irreversible monoamine oxidase type B (MAO-B) inhibitor (figure 6-7). In the brain, MAO-B is partly responsible for the catabolism of dopamine. Selegiline boosts the symptomatic effect of levodopa by slowing the breakdown of levodopa-derived dopamine in the brain. In the research literature selegiline was known as deprenyl or l-deprenyl. The standard dose is 5 mg with breakfast and lunch. Selegiline is absorbed and crosses the blood-brain barrier without difficulty. The serum half-lifes of selegiline and its meatbolites are less than 24 hours[71]. However, the clinical effect of selegiline may last months as loss of its effect is dependent on generation of new MAO-B in the brain.

How was selegiline created?

Selegiline was initially intended to be a "psychic energizer", created by combining an amphetamine moiety with an antidepressant-like compound[72]. The development of MAO inhibitors began in the 1950s, when iproniazid, an anti-tuberculosis agent, was found to improve depression. Early antidepressants were difficult to use as MAO-A inhibitors were associated with the risk of hypertensive crisis. Normally, MAO-A in the gut metabolizes ingested amines such as tyramine and prevents their absorption. When MAO-A in the gut is inhibited, ingested amines can be absorbed and may cause sympathomimetic crises, sometimes called the "cheese effect". Manifestations of sympathomimetic crisis include hypertension, vomiting, increased heart rate, and headache. When gut MAO-A is inhibited, levodopa can cause sympathomimetic crisis as readily as tyramine. For this reason, levodopa preparations should not be given concurrently with MAO-A inhibitors. As a relatively selective MAO-B inhibitor, selegiline can be safely administered with levodopa.

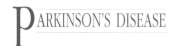

Selegiline is highly selective for inhibition of MAO-B in doses up to 10 mg per day [72]. Above 10 mg per day, it begins to lose its MAO-B selectivity and the risk of sympathomimetic crisis increases. Therefore, doses above 10 mg per day are generally not recommended.

What are the side-effects of selegiline?

Selegiline is generally well tolerated. It is typically administered in the morning and at midday rather than in the evening to minimize the potential for insomnia. Some patients experience gastrointestinal side-effects such as nausea [72]. When administered concurrently with levodopa, the most common side effect is an exacerbation of dopaminergic adverse effects. If a patient has peak-dose dyskinesias or hallucinations on levodopa, these may worsen with the addition of selegiline [73].

What medications should be avoided in patients who are taking selegiline?

A constellation of symptoms known as the serotonin syndrome may occur with the use of serotomimetic agents, taken alone or in combination with MAO inhibitors including selegiline. These agents include serotonin reuptake inhibitors, tricyclic and tetracyclic antidepressants, meperidine and other opiates, dextromethorphan, and tryptophan. The syndrome is characterized by various combinations of confusion, agitation, restlessness, rigidity, hyperreflexia, shivering, autonomic instability, myoclonus, coma, low grade fever, nausea, diarrhea, diaphoresis, flushing, and rarely rhabdomyolysis and death [74]. Patients taking selegiline should therefore avoid meperidine and other opiates.

The actual incidence of serious events when selegiline is used in combination with antidepressants is unknown. As many patients with Parkinson's disease suffer with depression, this issue raises difficult management questions. One chart review study did not identify any major side-effects from combination therapy and serious interactions appear to be rare [71,75].

When should I use selegiline?

Selegiline is beneficial as an adjunct to levodopa for patients who are experiencing deterioration in the quality of their response. For patients with motor fluctuations, selegiline reduces OFF time and extends the short duration response of levodopa. In addition, selegiline provides modest symptomatic benefit as monotherapy in early PD and can delay the need for other symptomatic treatments [76].

Why was there interest in whether selegiline could slow disease progression?

The concept that selegiline might slow disease progression initially came from three observations. The ability of the neurotoxin MPTP to cause dopamine cell death and induce parkinsonian symptoms in animals and man is dependent on its oxidation to MPP+ by MAO-B. When selegiline is administered prior to MPTP, MPTP is not converted to MPP+ and parkinsonian symptoms are not elicited [77]. If there is an environmental neurotoxin similar to MPTP that causes Parkinson's disease in man, then selegiline might prevent its oxidation and protect against dopamine cell damage. Similarly, if free radical formation from the oxidative metabolism of dopamine by MAO-B contributes to disease progression, inhibition of MAO-B by selegiline may reduce free radical formation and slow dopamine cell degeneration.

What is the DATATOP study?

The Parkinson Study Group examined the ability of selegiline and tocopherol (vitamin E), alone or together, to slow the progression of Parkinson's disease. This study was called "Deprenyl and Tocopherol Antioxidative Therapy of Parkinsonism", or DATATOP. Eight hundred patients with early Parkinson's disease not yet requiring levodopa therapy were enrolled in the study. Subjects were randomized to one of four groups: 1) selegiline (10 mg/day) and tocopherol placebo, 2) tocopherol (2000 IU/day) and selegiline placebo, 3) selegiline and tocopherol, or 4) selegiline placebo and tocopherol placebo. The primary endpoint was the time required for the patient to develop sufficient disability to warrant the use of levodopa therapy.

Results demonstrated that patients assigned to receive selegiline (alone or with tocopherol) experienced a significant delay in the need for levodopa therapy (hazard ratio = 0.50, p<0.001) (figure 6-8) [78]. Patients on selegiline placebo required levodopa at a projected median of 15 months from enrollment compared to 24 months for patients on selegiline. Tocopherol had no effect on the endpoint. This study demonstrates that the use of

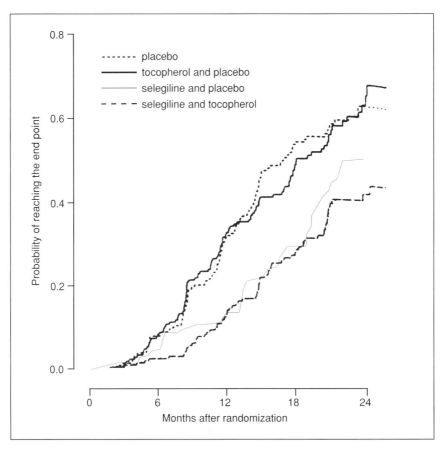

Figure 6-8. *DATATOP results. Kaplan-Meier estimate of the cumulative probability of reaching the end point, according to treatment group. The hazard ratio for patients assigned to selegiline compared to patients assigned to selegiline placebo with respect to the risk of reaching the end point per unit time is 0.50 (p<0.001; 95 percent confidence interval, 0.41 to 0.62).*

selegiline in early Parkinson's disease delays the need for levodopa therapy. However, the study also found that selegiline alone provided a small symptomatic benefit. One cannot exclude the possibility that the delay in need for levodopa was due entirely or in part to this small symptomatic effect.

What is the role of selegiline in the treatment of Parkinson's disease? Selegiline can be used in early Parkinson's disease to delay the need for levodopa and in advanced disease to decrease OFF time periods in patients with motor fluctuations. However, its symptomatic effects are generally modest.

What is rasagiline?

Rasagiline is a new MAO-B inhibitor that is currently in clinical testing. It provides symptomatic benefit in early disease when given as monotherapy [78b] and in advanced disease as an adjunct to levodopa in patients with motor fluctuations [78c]. There is interest in determining whether it can slow disease progression.

What are anticholinergic medications?

Anticholinergic medications were the mainstay of anti-parkinsonian treatment until the latter part of this century. They are most effective for reducing tremor [79], and usually provide minimal benefit with regard to bradykinesia and rigidity. In addition, tremor may or may not improve with anticholinergic agents and a given patient may respond to one anticholinergic but not others. Their use is often limited by side-effects and they are less well tolerated by older patients and those with dementia. Anticholinergics may cause confusion and hallucinations and most patients experience dry mouth or dry eyes [79]. Additional side-effects may include urinary retention, ocular accommodation abnormalities, abnormal sweating, and tachycardia. Anticholinergics should be used with caution in patients with glaucoma. The most commonly used anticholinergic medications are trihexyphenidyl-HCl (Artane®) and benztropine mesylate (Cogentin®).

What is amantadine?

Amantadine (Symmetrel®), or 1-amino-adamantine is an antiviral medication which was first found to improve symptoms in Parkinson's disease patients while being used to treat influenza in the 1960s. Subsequent trials confirmed that amantadine provides some benefit for the features of Parkinson's disease [80]. Interestingly, although amantadine provides only mild symptomatic benefit in early PD, when it is withdrawn from patients who have been on it for many years, there is often a dramatic worsening of PD symptoms [81]. Studies have demonstrated that amantadine can symptomatically reduce levodopa-induced peak-dose dyskinesias [82]. This effect has been shown to be maintained for at least one year [83].

Although amantadine's exact mechanism of action is unknown, it appears to augment dopamine release, may inhibit dopamine reuptake and may stimulate dopamine receptors[81]. Amantadine is well absorbed and has a long half-life of approximately 24 hours. It is usually administered at a dose of 100 mg BID or TID. Because of its urinary excretion, it should be used with caution in patients with renal disease. Amantadine is moderately well tolerated, and side-effects include hallucinations, confusion, nightmares, ankle edema, dry mouth, and livedo reticularis, an erythematous rash of the lower extremities. Hyponatremia has also been described. It can readily exacerbate hallucinations and should be used cautiously in patients with dementia.

CHAPTER 7

MEDICAL MANAGEMENT OF PARKINSON'S DISEASE

What is the goal of medical management of Parkinson's disease?

The goal of medical management of Parkinson's disease is to adequately control signs and symptoms while minimizing side-effects for as long as possible.

What are some general guidelines for the use of medications in Parkinson's disease?

It is recommended to make only one medication change at a time so that the positive and negative effects of that change are clear.

Symptomatic medications should be initiated at a low dose and slowly escalated based on clinical response in order to minimize the incidence of early side-effects. Signs and symptoms progress slowly and rapid medication changes are rarely required.

Although knowledge and experience are useful guides, each patient must be assessed and treated as an individual.

Will medications eliminate the signs and symptoms of Parkinson's disease? Except in very early disease, medications will not entirely eliminate signs and symptoms of Parkinson's disease. As the disease progresses, symptoms increase despite best medical management. Asymmetry often persists with worse signs apparent in the first-affected extremity.

How do I know if an increase in medication is warranted?

The presence of functional disability warrants a trial of increased medication therapy. Experience is the best guide to realistic expectations. Nonetheless, if symptom control is inadequate, an attempt to bring about

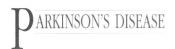

improvement is warranted. If no improvement can be achieved before intolerable side-effects emerge, the lowest medication dose that will maintain the current level of function is appropriate.

What is the general approach to the medical treatment of Parkinson's disease?

One attempts to provide adequate symptomatic control throughout the course of the disease. The younger and healthier the patient, the more aggressively we base our treatment on strategies designed to maximize function over the long term. This includes the use of dopamine agonist monotherapy prior to the use of levodopa and consideration of introducing entacapone when levodopa is first introduced. These strategies provide more continuous dopamine receptor stimulation. Studies in PD patients have demonstrated that initiation of dopamine therapy with a dopamine agonist causes less motor fluctuations and dyskinesia than levodopa alone. The addition of entacapone at the time levodopa is inroduced has been demonstrated to cause less motor fluctuations and dyskinesia in the MPTP monkey model of PD. These approaches can be easily implemented without compromising symptomatic control.

When should one introduce symptomatic medication therapy for Parkinson's disease?

Symptomatic medications are generally initiated when the patient begins to experience functional disability. Patients with very early disease should be monitored clinically for the development of functional disability.

What is functional disability?

Functional disability is present when symptoms of Parkinson's disease interfere with activities the patient either wants or needs to do. This should be assessed individually for each patient in the context of his/her lifestyle. A small loss of finger dexterity may threaten a keyboard operator's livelihood and warrant symptomatic therapy, whereas a retiree may have greater motor dysfunction without disability and may not require symptomatic therapy.

What should I do when a patient develops functional disability?

Symptomatic therapy should be initiated when functional disability emerges. For many patients, especially those with younger-onset of symptoms, we begin symptomatic therapy with a dopamine agonist. Dopamine agonists provide anti-parkinsonian benefit approximately equal to levodopa therapy for six months to a year and may adequately control symptoms for several years. Levodopa is added when agonist therapy alone no longer provides sufficient symptomatic benefit. By starting symptomatic therapy with a dopamine agonist one delays the need for levodopa and provides relatively smooth dopamine receptor stimulation. Once levodopa therapy becomes necessary, one is able to use lower doses when it is administered concurrently with an agonist. There is good evidence to suggest that this approach is associated with a lower prevalence of dyskinesia[1-4]. One can then consider whether entacapone should be added as soon as levodopa therapy is introduced in order to continue to provide relatively smoother dopamine stimulation. An equivalent alternative is the use of levodopa/carbidopa/entacapone for the initiation of levodopa therapy This approach has been suggested by monkey studies but has not been proven in patients.

For older-onset patients and those with dementia, more emphasis is placed on short term considerations and one may elect to use levodopa rather than dopamine agonists as the first symptomatic agent. We use the lowest levodopa dosage that will adequately control symptoms. One may also elect to use levodopa as the first symptomatic agent for patients who are very immobile, bradykinetic or rigid, and for those who require relatively rapid improvement. In these cases, a dopamine agonist can then be introduced shortly thereafter when reasonable control of parkinsonian symptoms has been achieved.

How do you dose the dopamine agonists?

The agonists are best introduced at a low dose and slowly escalated. Reasonably high doses should be achieved before their utility is assessed. An opportunity for improvement may be lost if they are judged ineffective at low doses. The two most commonly used dopamine agonists are ropinirole and pramipexole. Ropinirole is commonly initiated at 0.25 mg TID for one week, 0.50 mg TID for the second week, 0.75 TID for the third week, 1.0 mg TID for the fourth week, 1.5 mg TID for the fifth week, 2 mg TID for the sixth week, 2.5 mg TID for the seventh week and 3.0 mg TID for the eighth week. Further dose adjustments are made at increments of 0.50 mg TID per week based on patient response up to a maximum recommended dose of 24 mg per day. Pramipexole is initiated at 0.125 mg TID for one week, 0.25 TID for the second week, and 0.50 TID the third week. Further dose adjustments are made in increments of 0.25 TID per week based on patient response up to a maximum recommended dose of 1.5 mg TID.

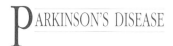

What should I do when dopamine agonist monotherapy no longer provides adequate symptomatic control?

Levodopa therapy is generally required when dopamine agonist monotherapy no longer provides adequate symptomatic control. The dopamine agonist can be continued and levodopa added. This may reduce the long term incidence of motor complications [2-4]. In addition, less levodopa is required, levodopa-induced free radical formation may be diminished, and dopamine receptors are buffered from fluctuating concentrations of levodopa-derived dopamine.

What is the role of COMT inhibitors?

COMT inhibitors extend the peripheral half-life of levodopa and increase its central bioavailability. Entacapone can be considered when levodopa is first introduced in an effort to reduce the long term emergence of motor fluctuations and dyskinesia. In advanced patients with motor fluctuations on levodopa, COMT inhibitors reduce OFF time and improve motor function. The strategy of smoothing dopamine receptor stimulation can be maximized with the concurrent administration of a COMT inhibitor and a dopamine agonist as adjuncts to levodopa.

What levodopa formulation should I use when levodopa therapy is first required?

Standard levodopa/carbidopa, levodopa/carbidopa ER, and levodopa/carbidopa/entacapone are equally effective in improving motor symptoms when levodopa is first required. Generic formulations of standard and ER levodopa/carbidopa are available and are less expensive than the brand formulations. Patients find the levodopa/carbidopa ER or levodopa/carbidopa/entacapone formulations more convenient because fewer daily doses may be required. There is interest as to whether more continuous dopamine receptor stimulation as afforded by levodopa/carbidopa/entacapone can forestall the development of long term complications including motor fluctuations and dyskinesia.

How do I dose levodopa?

It is helpful to introduce levodopa at a low dose and then escalate slowly to minimize the incidence of side-effects. Standard carbidopa/levodopa can be introduced at a dose of one half of a 25/100 tablet per day and escalated to a target of either one half tablet QID or one tablet TID over one month. For carbidopa/levodopa ER, the initial target dose is 25/100 TID or 50/200 BID, usually starting with 100 mg levodopa per day and slowly increasing over a period of one to three weeks.

Levodopa/carbidopa/entacapone, when used as initial levodopa therapy, is usually initiated at a dose of one 50/12.5/200 mg tablet (50 mg levodopa) or one 100/25/200 mg tablet (100 mg levodopa) per day and increased by one tablet a day each week to a TID or QID schedule. Further escalations are undertaken based on clinical response.

What is the usual timeline for this long term strategy?

There is a lot of variability in the rate of progression of Parkinson's disease. Nonetheless, most patients will require symptomatic therapy within one to two years of symptom onset. Once functional disability emerges, a dopamine agonist will often control symptoms for another one to four years before levodopa is required.

How much levodopa is too much?

Most experts try to keep the levodopa dose below 500-600 mg per day for as long as possible. Despite this, patients should receive as much levodopa as is necessary to adequately control symptoms. If the patient has sufficient bradykinesia and rigidity to cause meaningful disability, the levodopa dose should be increased. There is no maximal levodopa dose, and some patients require relatively high doses (~1000 - 1500 mg levodopa or more) to achieve good benefit. At some point in a levodopa escalation, the patient will encounter an intolerable side effect and this defines "too much" levodopa for that patient. If the levodopa dose is escalated and no additional benefit occurs, the dose should be tapered down to the lowest dose that still provides the current level of benefit. Higher levodopa dosages that do not bring about additional benefit should be avoided.

What does it mean if there is no improvement when I add levodopa?

Almost all Parkinson's disease patients with sufficient bradykinesia and rigidity will experience improvement when levodopa therapy is introduced. There are several reasons why there may be no appreciable response. The dose may be too low, the diagnosis may be wrong,

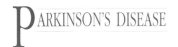

attention may be focused on the wrong symptoms, or symptoms may be so slight that improvement is hard to identify. Most Parkinson's disease patients experience noticeable improvement with 600 mg of levodopa per day or less. Much of this improvement is reduced bradykinesia and rigidity, and increased mobility and dexterity. If no improvement is noted, and symptoms remain prominent, the dose should be slowly escalated to tolerance or at least 1000 mg per day.

Improvement in bradykinesia and rigidity may be overlooked if too much attention is focused on tremor. Tremor may or may not respond to levodopa. If the patient has minimal difficulty with bradykinesia, rigidity, dexterity and mobility, improvement may be hard to detect. Patients with atypical parkinsonism usually do not benefit from levodopa therapy.

Patients who have been on levodopa for some time may be unaware of the benefit that it is providing. If there is a question as to whether levodopa is providing benefit, a temporary taper is often helpful.

How should I approach the treatment of tremor?

Tremor usually does not cause much functional disability in Parkinson's disease. We attempt to treat bradykinesia and rigidity with dopaminergic medications and then evaluate residual tremor. If a functionally disabling tremor persists or is the only manifestation of Parkinson's disease, an anticholinergic medication can be introduced. Tremor is variably responsive to levodopa, dopamine agonists and anticholinergic medications. In addition, tremor may respond to one anticholinergic but not another, so it is worth trying several (sequentially) if necessary. Patients with medically refractory, disabling tremor may benefit from a surgical procedure such as deep brain stimulation.

What if my patient can't tolerate levodopa?

The long term treatment of Parkinson's disease without levodopa is almost always less than satisfactory. When a patient has disabling parkinsonian symptoms it is very important to employ all conceivable strategies to try to achieve tolerability. Smaller doses than were previously used should be employed to reintroduce the medication. If necessary, a levodopa tablet can be crushed and one small chip per day used as the starting dose. If a patient has difficulty initiating levodopa therapy due to nausea, he should be instructed to take it immediately following a meal. If nausea persists, additional carbidopa or benserazide may be helpful.

Although 75 mg of carbidopa per day is usually sufficient to saturate peripheral decarboxylase, some patients will benefit from carbidopa in doses up to 200 mg per day. In some cases, a peripheral dopamine blocker such as domperidone will be required, and this is usually quite effective. For patients whose intolerability is due to orthostatic hypotension, fludrocortisone or midodrine may be beneficial.

How can I treat motor fluctuations?

After several years of a stable response through the day, many patients on levodopa begin to experience motor fluctuations and notice that the benefit wears off after a few hours. It is usually relatively easy to reduce OFF time in a patient with motor fluctuations who is not experiencing peak-dose dyskinesia. Several different strategies, alone or in combination, can be used to provide more sustained dopaminergic therapy. Possible strategies include adding selegiline, a dopamine agonist, or a COMT inhibitor, dosing levodopa more frequently, increasing the levodopa dose, switching from standard to a long-acting preparation or levodopa/carbidopa/entacapone (figure 7-1). The patient should be alerted to the fact that increased dopaminergic therapy may cause or worsen peak-dose dyskinesia.

How do I manage patients with both motor fluctuations and dyskinesia?

Patients with both motor fluctuations and troublesome peak-dose dyskinesia can present a difficult management challenge. The goal of treatment for these patients is to provide as much good functional time through the day as possible. This is accomplished by maximizing ON time without troublesome dyskinesia. An attempt is made to reduce both OFF time and troublesome or disabling dyskinesia. An increase in dopaminergic therapy may increase dyskinesia and a decrease in dopaminergic therapy may increase OFF time. For many patients with severe fluctuations and dyskinesia, the best that can be done with medications is to balance OFF time and dyskinesia. The patient's relative preference for OFF time versus dyskinesia should be taken into account.

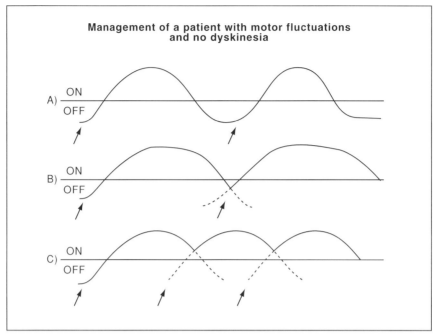

Figure 7-1. *Management of a patient with motor fluctuations and no dyskinesia (A). Off time can be reduced by using a higher levodopa dose (B), switching to a long acting preparation (B), adding a dopamine agonist, COMT inhibitor or selegiline (B), or by shortening the interdose interval (C). Arrows indicate times of levodopa administration.*

Improvement is sought by attempting to provide as stable dopaminergic stimulation as possible within the therapeutic target zone. The addition of selegiline, a dopamine agonist, or a COMT inhibitor may be helpful. Dyskinesia may increase when these medications are added and downward titration of levodopa should then be undertaken. For patients on extended release levodopa preparations it is often helpful to switch to a standard levodopa preparation to provide a more consistent and predictable dosing cycle (figure 7-2). It is then critical to titrate the dose based on clinical response.

In general, it is desirable to administer smaller levodopa doses more frequently. A dose should be sought which is sufficient to turn the patient on without causing too much dyskinesia (figure 7-3). The time to wearing-off then determines the appropriate interdose interval. Ideally, the next dose should be given to take effect when the previous dose begins to wear off. This can then be refined by the addition of a dopamine agonist, COMT inhibitor, or selegiline, with possible additional titration of the levodopa dose, to further smooth the clinical response. In advanced disease, if a

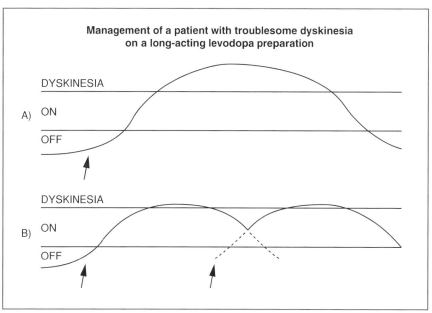

Figure 7-2. *Patients with troublesome dyskinesia while on a long-acting levodopa preparation (A) may benefit from a switch to standard levodopa/PDI (B). This may allow for better titration and a more consistent dosing cycle. Arrows indicate times of levodopa administration.*

patient's response has become extremely erratic, he may have to take his next levodopa dose when he feels the previous dose wearing off rather than adhering to a fixed dosing schedule. When medication is no longer effective in the management of motor fluctuations and dyskinesia, deep brain stimulation should be considered.

Does diet play a role in motor fluctuations?

Levodopa competes with other large neutral amino acids for transport across the blood-brain barrier. Protein ingested in meals can slow levodopa flow into the brain. This usually has no impact on patients with relatively early disease, but can have a dramatic effect on patients with more advanced disease as clinical status becomes critically dependent on continuous levodopa transport into the brain. Patients with severe fluctuations and those who find they turn off following a meal may benefit from a low protein or protein redistributed diet[6]. In addition, balanced carbohydrate-protein commercial food preparations are available. For patients with severe motor fluctuations, minimizing serum protein fluctuations may reduce the variability of levodopa transport and help provide a more stable clinical response.

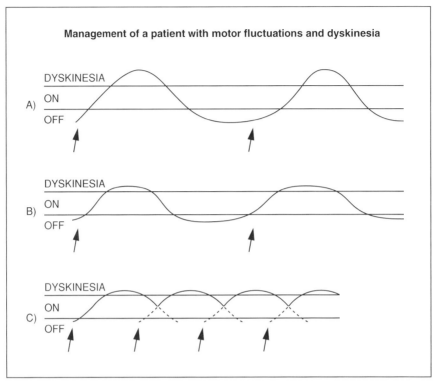

Figure 7-3. *The treatment of patients with motor fluctuations and peak-dose dyskinesia (A) generally involves providing less levodopa more frequently. The levodopa dose should be lowered until it brings on only mild dyskinesia (B). The time to wearing off then determines the interdose interval (C). Arrows indicate times of levodopa administration.*

How can I make levodopa take effect faster?

For patients with motor fluctuations, standard levodopa formulations commonly take 20-30 minutes or more before an effect is apparent. By chewing the tablet, the absorption rate is increased and clinical benefit occurs more rapidly. Another option is to dissolve the tablet in orange juice. This may be particularly useful for patients taking levodopa on an as needed basis when the previous dose has worn off and for patients who awaken immobile at night and need symptomatic benefit as quickly as possible.

What is liquid levodopa?

Patients with severe fluctuations and dyskinesia may gain some benefit when placed on a "liquid levodopa" regimen[7]. Patients are instructed to dissolve ten standard carbidopa/levodopa 25/100 tablets in one liter of water with one-half teaspoon of ascorbic acid. The result is a one mg per milliliter levodopa solution. The solution should be made fresh every day and hourly dosing is usually employed. An initial dosing schedule is calculated and further adjustments must be made to titrate to clinical response.

The first dose of the day is the same as had been taken in pill form. Initial hourly doses are calculated by dividing the patient's prior daily levodopa dose by the number of hourly doses he will be taking. When possible, the first daily dose is adjusted before the hourly doses. Adjustments are made in 5 mg increments every three to five days. Rather precise measurements are required for consistent dosing and many patients use a syringe to measure each dose. For successful initiation of liquid therapy it is critical to inform patients that the initial recommended schedule is only a rough guess as to dosing.

The ultimate benefit of a liquid regimen can only be assessed after optimal titration, which usually takes several weeks. Without this warning patients are likely to abandon liquid therapy in the first few days when they experience increased off time or dyskinesia. Aggressive titration is vital. Most patients on liquid therapy use the levodopa solution through the day and take a carbidopa/levodopa ER tablet at bedtime to help them get through the night.

Most patients find the liquid levodopa regimen rather cumbersome and abandon it after some time.

What is the role of amantadine in patients with motor fluctuations and dyskinesias?

Amantadine may be beneficial in reducing OFF time and has also been shown to significantly improve dyskinesia [8]. Amantadine is initiated at a dose of 100 mg BID and can be escalated up to 400 mg daily.

How do I treat wearing-off dystonia?

Wearing-off dystonia often responds to more sustained dopaminergic therapy. Substantial improvement is usually brought about by the addition of a dopamine agonist. Some patients benefit from a bedtime dose of a long acting levodopa preparation and/or the addition of a COMT inhibitor.

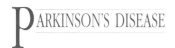

How do I treat diphasic dyskinesia?

Diphasic dyskinesia can be difficult to treat. In general, an attempt is made to increase and smooth dopaminergic stimulation. The goal is to avoid turning on and wearing-off as much as possible since these are the phases of the dosing cycle in which diphasic dyskinesia occurs. If medical therapy is not benefical, deep brain stimulation should be considered.

What should I do if my patient is confused?

Dementia occurs in approximately 15-30% of Parkinson's disease patients [9]. It typically occurs late in the disease and progresses over time. Confusion can be exacerbated by medications. If confusion is present a review of all of the patient's medications is in order to identify those that are particularly associated with confusion. Any unnecessary medications should be discontinued. Any of the anti-parkinsonian medications can cause or exacerbate confusion. If confusion is evident, anti-parkinsonian medications should be reduced to see if improvement can be achieved.

One might first reduce and eliminate anticholinergics, amantadine and then selegiline followed by reducing and eliminating the dopamine agonists. If necessary, the levodopa dose can be reduced. Patients with confusion may respond to medications used for Alzheimer's disease such as donepezil (Aricept®), rivastigmine (Exelon®), and galantamine (Reminyl®).

What should I do if my patient experiences hallucinations?

One must evaluate the impact of hallucinations. If the hallucinations are mild and non-bothersome, no change may be necessary. An attempt should be made to alleviate more severe hallucinations. Amantadine and anticholinergics, and if necessary, the dopamine agonists can be discontinued. The levodopa dose can be decreased to see if hallucinations can be ameliorated while still maintaining control of motor symptoms. If motor fluctuations are present, levodopa plus a COMT inhibitor may be the most useful combination.

If a satisfactory balance between motor symptom control and hallucinations cannot be achieved by titrating levodopa, consideration is given to adding an atypical neuroleptic. Classical neuroleptics such as haloperidol reduce hallucinations but worsen motor symptoms. The preferred treatment is an atypical neuroleptic with minimal parkinsonian side-effects. Quetiapine (Seroquel®) and Clozapine (Clozaril®) are useful to reduce hallucinations and have minimal parkinsonian side-effects[10,11].

The most common side effect of clozapine is hypotension. The main serious side effect is the risk of neutropenia. Because of this risk, weekly monitoring of the patient's white blood cell count is required. The doses used to treat hallucinations in Parkinson's disease are much lower than those used to treat schizophrenia. Therapy can be initiated with one quarter of a 25 mg tablet at bedtime and slowly escalated every two to three days by one quarter tablet until a beneficial dose is achieved. Most patients experience benefit at a dose of 25-75 mg per day.

Quetiapine is another atypical neuroleptic with minimal parkinsonian side-effects[11]. It has become the treatment of choice for hallucinations in PD because it is not associated with agranulocytosis and blood monitoring is not required. Quetiapine is initiated at a dose of 25 mg at bedtime and escalated every two to three days by 25 mg until a benefical dose is reached. The usual dosing range is 25-300 mg per day.

Fernandez et al. treated PD patients with drug-induced psychosis with quetiapine at a mean dose of 40.6 mg/day[12]. Twenty of the 24 Parkinson's disease patients who had never received a neuroleptic showed marked improvement in psychosis without worsening of motor symptoms.

Clozapine and quetiapine are quite effective in reducing hallucinations but do not improve underlying dementia.

How can I treat Atypical Parkinsonism?

Anti-parkinsonian medications usually do not provide meaningful benefit for the clinical features of Atypical Parkinsonisms. Nonetheless, one can perform a levodopa trial, introducing it at a low dose and slowly escalating until intolerable side-effects emerge. The goal is to achieve a levodopa dose of at least 1000 - 1500 mg to be satisfied that an adequate trial has been completed. If no benefit is realized, taper the dose downward to see if a loss of symptomatic benefit can be identified. When benefit occurs it is usually modest and fleeting. Medication is discontinued if no benefit is identified. One of the reasons to perform a levodopa trial is to be sure not to misdiagnose an unusual presentation of Parkinson's disease and miss an opportunity for improvement. Much of the management of Atypical Parkinsonisms is supportive. Secondary symptoms such as depression and constipation should be identified and treated.

CHAPTER 8

MANAGEMENT OF NON-MOTOR SYMPTOMS OF PARKINSON'S DISEASE

How should I approach depression in Parkinson's disease?

Depression is the most common mood disturbance in Parkinson's disease, affecting roughly 40 to 50% of patients[1]. Parkinson's disease patients experience major depression more frequently than the normal elderly, and are significantly more depressed than nonparkinsonian control patients with comparable disability[2]. Depressed Parkinson's disease patients often meet clinical criteria for either major depression or dysthymic disorder[2,3] and often have concurrent symptoms of panic and anxiety[4]. Most studies have not found an association between depression in Parkinson's disease and severity or duration of illness, age, or gender[5]. In general, Parkinson's disease patients have less self-blame and guilt than their depressed, nonparkinsonian counterparts[6].

It is unclear whether the etiology of depression in Parkinson's disease is endogenous, reactive, or both. There is evidence that depression in Parkinson's disease is related to serotonergic abnormalities[7]. Nonetheless, it appears likely that both neurochemical changes and psychosocial issues may contribute to the development of depression in Parkinson's disease.

Antidepressants have been found to improve depression in Parkinson's disease patients in a limited number of studies[8-10]. Tricyclic antidepressants, serotonin reuptake inhibitors, and atypical antidepressants have all been found to improve depression in Parkinson's disease patients. However, several case reports have noted worsening of parkinsonian symptoms after treatment with the serotonin reuptake inhibitors fluoxetine (Prozac®) and paroxetine (Paxil®)[11,12]. An open label study of sertraline (Zoloft®) found it to reduce depression in stable Parkinson's disease patients without worsening motor symptoms[13].

Patients who experience depressed mood only when levodopa wears off may benefit from strategies that smooth dopamine replacement therapy and may not require an antidepressants.

What is the serotonin syndrome?

Selective serotonin reuptake inhibitors (SSRI's) are commonly used to treat depression in Parkinson's disease. However, SSRI's, either alone or in combination with monoamine oxidase inhibitors such as selegiline, can cause the "serotonin syndrome", characterized by mental status changes, tremor, diaphoresis, and incoordination. Deaths have occurred due to rhabdomyolysis, disseminated intravascular coagulation, respiratory distress syndrome, and cardiovascular collapse [14-16]. Treatment of the serotonin syndrome involves discontinuation of the inciting drug and supportive measures, with resolution of symptoms usually occurring in hours to weeks [17].

The occurrence of serotonin syndrome in Parkinson's disease patients receiving both selegiline and SSRI's is rare. A retrospective chart review evaluating the concomitant use of fluoxetine and selegiline failed to uncover any serious side-effects or additional adverse events which had not already been reported with each medication alone [18]. A survey of physicians in the Parkinson Study Group (PSG) indicates that the combined use of selegiline and antidepressants rarely results in serious adverse events [19].

How do I treat orthostatic hypotension?

Orthostatic hypotension is defined as a drop of 30 mm Hg in systolic blood pressure or a drop of 20 mm Hg in mean blood pressure (diastolic plus one third of the pulse pressure) when going from the supine to standing position. Patients usually complain of lightheadedness and if the orthostatic hypotension is severe syncope can occur. Asymptomatic orthostatic hypotension does not require intervention but patients whose blood pressure is no higher than 80/50 mm Hg are usually symptomatic. Associated symptoms include syncope and presyncope but they may also be non-specific such as fatigue, unsteadiness, headache, neck tightness or cognitive slowing, especially in the elderly.

As a first step, unnecessary medications should be discontinued. The patient should drink eight or more glasses of fluid each day and liberally add salt (up to 150-250 mEq) to the diet. Pharmacologic treatment can be undertaken to increase intravascular volume with mineralocorticoids [20], or to increase vascular resistance through stimulation of alpha receptors [21,22]. The mineralocorticoid fludrocortisone (Florinef®) is introduced at a dose of 0.1 mg once or twice a day and can be increased to as high as 0.3 to 0.6 mg per day. Supine hypertension and dependent edema are common and not unexpected but care must be taken to avoid congestive heart failure.

Midodrine (ProAmatine®) is a peripherally acting alpha-1-agonist that produces vasoconstriction of both arterioles and venous capacitance vessels [23,24]. The initial recommended dosage is 2.5 mg BID or TID. The usual maintenance dose is 30 mg/day in divided doses, with a maximum of 40 mg/day. It is well absorbed orally and generally well tolerated. Side-effects include scalp pruritus and tingling, pilomotor reactions, gastrointestinal complaints, headache, and dizziness [23]. Because it does not cross the blood-brain barrier, it is less likely to produce central nervous system side-effects than ephedrine [24]. As a selective alpha-adrenergic agonist, it is relatively free of beta-adrenergic side-effects and pulse rate usually does not increase [23]. Patients with supine hypertension on midodrine (>150/90) should be treated by elevating the head of the bed to a 30 degree incline.

Several open label and double-blind studies have shown that midodrine effectively controls symptoms of orthostatic hypotension in most patients [21,26]. Refractory cases may respond to combination therapy with fludrocortisone and midodrine [22]. Rarely, ergotamine tartrate (Cafergot) is used in the treatment of orthostatic hypotension.

What is the treatment of constipation in Parkinson's disease?

Constipation is common in Parkinson's disease. In a study comparing colonic transit time between Parkinson's disease patients and age and sex-matched controls, Parkinson's disease patients had delayed colonic transit affecting all segments of the colon [27]. Additional studies have identified decreased basal anal sphincter pressures and a hyper-contractile external sphincter response [28-30].

Colonic abnormalities in Parkinson's disease may have both central and peripheral causes. Lewy bodies have been found in the myenteric plexus of the colon, suggesting that Parkinson's disease may affect the enteric nervous system. There is also a report of the presence of Lewy bodies in the neurons of the dorsal group of the nucleus intermediolateralis of the

3rd sacral segment of the spinal cord (31). Anismus, or paradoxical contraction of the striated sphincter muscles during defecation, may be part of a focal dystonia. Administration of apomorphine has resulted in improved defecation, suggesting that these problems may be related to dopamine deficiency[32].

Basic treatment of constipation is aimed at increasing stool bulk by adding more fiber to the diet and by increasing daily liquid intake. Fiber intake can be increased by having the patient eat more fruits and raw vegetables, as well as products containing bran. Exercise may also be helpful in alleviating constipation. Anticholinergics that inhibit gastric motility and promote GI dryness should be discontinued. Despite these measures, many patients still complain of significant straining and hard stools. Stool softeners such as docusate sodium (Colace®) may be necessary.

Polyethylene glycol (Miralax®) is an osmotic agent that causes water to be retained with the stool. It softens the stool and increases the frequency of bowel movements. The usual dose is 17 grams (one heaping tablespoon) of powder per day in eight ounces of water, soda, or juice.

For patients with refractory constipation, lactulose preparations may be required. When possible, the long term use of pharmacologic agents in treating constipation should be avoided. The simplest measures are best tolerated long term.

How can I treat drooling?

It is estimated that 70% of Parkinson's disease patients eventually experience drooling[33]. Siallorhea in Parkinson's disease is caused by saliva pooling in the mouth secondary to swallowing difficulties, rather than from increased production of saliva[34]. Besides being bothersome to the patient, siallorhea can lead to more serious problems including chemical dermatitis or aspiration.

For some patients, increased dopaminergic therapy is useful to improve swallowing and reduce drooling. Anticholinergic medications can reduce saliva production, but may cause side-effects including dry mouth, constipation, and cognitive changes. The peripheral anticholinergic glycopyrrolate (Robinul®) may be particularly useful to avoid cognitive side-effects. More recently, injections of botulinum toxin into salivary glands have been described as an effective treatment for drooling. For the most difficult cases, salivary duct sclerosis may be considered.

How can I treat dysphagia?

Dysphagia is also common in Parkinson's disease and patients often describe a "choking" sensation along with difficulty swallowing foods. Parkinson's disease can cause esophageal dysfunction and abnormalities in the oropharyngeal phase of swallowing. In one study of swallowing disorders in asymptomatic elderly patients with Parkinson's disease, videofluoroscopy was performed to evaluate facial, tongue, and palatopharyngeal musculature [35]. Although these patients denied any dysphagic symptoms, all patients had at least one abnormality of the swallowing mechanism. Oropharyngeal transit time was increased and patients needed more swallows to remove the bolus from the pharynx.

Lewy bodies have been found in the myenteric plexus in the esophagus in dysphagic Parkinson's disease patients [36], again suggesting that the enteric nervous system is affected. Radionucleotide motility studies have revealed slow transit time and demonstrated that dysphagia may improve with antiparkinson medication [37]. Dysphagia may increase the risk of aspiration, although one study failed to demonstrate increased rates of pulmonary infection in Parkinson's disease patients with dysphagia [58].

Parkinson's disease patients with dysphagia should eliminate hard foods from the diet and pay careful attention to swallowing. Increased dopaminergic therapy with levodopa may improve swallowing [39]. For patients with clinically significant dysphagia it is worthwhile to slowly increase the levodopa dose to tolerance to evaluate whether any improvement in dysphagia can be achieved.

How should I approach urinary incontinence in Parkinson's disease? Patients complaining of urinary symptoms should have a urologic evaluation including cystometric studies to exclude other causes of urinary symptoms, including prostate abnormalities. Decreased levels of dopamine can cause detrusor hyperreflexia in Parkinson's disease patients, resulting in urinary frequency, urgency, and most commonly nocturia. A high incidence of instability of the detrusor muscles has been reported in incontinent Parkinson's disease patients [40].

A simple reduction in fluids after dinner may help to reduce nocturia [40]. Otherwise, use of an anticholinergic medication such as tolterodine tartrate (Detrol®, Detrol LA®), oxybutinin chloride (Ditropan®, Ditropan XL®) or

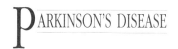

propantheline bromide (Pro-Banthine®, Propanthel®) may be helpful. Tolterodine long acting is given in dosages of 4 mg once a day and the immediate release is given in dosages of 2 mg twice a day, oxybutinin is given in dosages of 5 to 10 mg at bedtime, and propantheline is administered in dosages of 15 to 30 mg at bedtime. Patients should be monitored for cognitive side-effects. Of these medications, tolterodine is least likely to cause cognitive side-effects.

If detrusor hypoactivity is present, a reduction in anticholinergic medications may be warranted. The use of desmopressin nasal spray to treat nocturia in Parkinson's disease has been explored. It may be considered for patients with significant adverse impact due to nocturia refractory to other measures [41] as electrolyte imbalance is a possible side effect.

How should I approach sexual dysfunction in Parkinson's disease? Sexual dysfunction can occur for a variety of reasons including lack of mobility, loss of interest, or difficulty achieving and maintaining erection. Nonetheless, the exact pathophysiology of sexual dysfunction is largely unknown. Loss of sexual interest is commonly reported in Parkinson's disease patients, and both men and women are affected. However, one study suggested that loss of sexual interest, although common, is no greater than that which occurs in other non-neurologic chronic diseases [42]. Depression and use of medications such as propranolol and other antihypertensives can contribute to sexual dysfunction [43,44]. After discontinuation of potentially offending medications and treatment of depression, a patient complaining of sexual dysfunction should be evaluated by a urologist to exclude other causes and direct further management.

Sildenafil citrate (Viagra®) is a phosphodiesterase type V inhibitor used to treat erectile dysfunction, and studies are being conducted to evaluate its safety and efficacy in treating erectile dysfunction in PD. In one open-label study of sildenafil citrate use in men with PD and erectile dysfunction, there were significant improvements in total Sexual Health Inventory Scores, overall sexual satisfaction, satisfaction with sexual desire, ability to achieve erection, ability to maintain an erection, and ability to reach orgasm [45]. No changes were noted in motor function with sildenafil citrate use.

How should I treat seborrhea?

It is not uncommon to find excessive oiliness, chafing and redness of the skin, particularly of the forehead and scalp, in Parkinson's disease patients. Dandruff shampoos containing salicylic acid and coal tars can help with itching and flaking. Hydrocortisone cream 1% can be obtained over-the-counter and can be helpful if applied to the scalp or affected skin areas once or twice daily. Ketoconazole (Nizoral®) is available as a prescription cream or shampoo and can be helpful in some cases. The cream is applied to the skin twice daily for up to four weeks and the shampoo is used twice weekly for four weeks. If clinically warranted, the use of topical steroids may be beneficial. If there is an inadequate response, referral to a dermatologist for further evaluation and treatment is appropriate.

How can I treat postural instability (imbalance)?

There is no medication therapy that is known to be effective to treat true balance dysfunction. However, there are multiple reasons why a patient with Parkinson's disease may be prone to falls. If a patient is falling because of poor mobility or shortened gait, improvement may occur with increased levodopa therapy. In addition, the patient's neurologic status should be carefully reviewed to determine if any non-Parkinson's disease signs are contributing to falls. This might include sensory dysfunction that might be amenable to treatment, and weakness that might be the result of stroke or other neurologic disorders.

In general, the approach to postural instability is to try to keep the patient active but safe. Some patients benefit from the use of a three-wheeled walker with hand brakes, and some may benefit from physical therapy. Unfortunately, these are only temporizing measures as postural instability is likely to progress once present.

How Can I Treat Sleep Difficulties in Parkinson's Disease?

There are multiple causes of sleep difficulties in Parkinson's disease patients. Some sleep problems can be managed through the use of "sleep hygiene", or good sleep habits. This includes a consistent sleep schedule, reduction of daytime napping, regular physical exercise, reduction of stimulant use such as caffeine at nighttime and a healthy diet. A careful review of all current medications is important as Parkinson's disease patients are often taking several medications that can affect sleep.

If nighttime awakenings are related to parkinsonian symptoms such as reduced movement, tremor, or dystonia, the use of extended release levodopa, Stalevo, COMT inhibitors, or dopamine agonists at bedtime can be helpful. If the patient awakens and night and cannot get back to sleep because he is OFF, a standard levodopa formulation dissolved in orange juice or chewed and swallowed may provide relief after some time.

Vivid dreams and visual hallucinations can also lead to sleep problems. The addition of quetiapine (Seroquel®) in dosages of 25-100 mg at bedtime can help with these problems. Depression and anxiety commonly occur in Parkinson's disease and can affect sleep. If patients have depression or anxiety, the addition of an antidepressant or an anxiolytic can improve sleep quality. Some sleep problems may be related to nocturia. In these cases, the use of medications such as tolterodine (Detrol®, Detrol LA®) at bedtime can be helpful to reduce bladder spasms.

Sleep disorders such as periodic limb movements in sleep (PLMS) and sleep apnea increase in incidence with age. PD patients may also have rapid eye movement (REM) behavior disorder (RBD). Patients with RBD or PLMS may benefit from the use of clonazepam (Klonopin®) in dosages of 0.5-2 mg at bedtime. In patients with sleep apnea, sleep studies and the use of continuous positive airway pressure (CPAP) should be attempted.

Finally, in some patients the use of hypnotics may be the only way to treat insomnia. In patients with difficulty falling asleep the use of short acting hypnotics such as zolpidem (Ambien®) or zaleplon (Sonata®) should be tried. In patients with difficulty staying asleep, longer acting agents like trazadone (Desyrel®), mirtazapine (Remeron®) or temazepam (Restoril®) can be helpful, but hangover effects may cause drowsiness or falls in the morning.

How do I treat sleepiness in PD?

Excessive daytime sleepiness (EDS) in PD can potentially be caused by the disease itself, insomnia, sleep disorders, or medications. A careful history may help pinpoint a particular cause. Medications should be carefully reviewed to identify those that might be causing sleepiness. These can be reduced or discontinued if feasible. Dopamine agonists and other dopaminergic medications including levodopa can cause sleepiness and this should be considered. If no obvious cause for sleepiness is identified, an overnight sleep test (polysomnogram) should be considered in an effort to diagnose possible sleep apnea or other sleep disorders.

Modafinil (Provigil®) is a wake-promoting agent that is effective to reduce EDS in narcolepsy. Preliminary information suggests that it is also effective to reduce sleepiness in PD [46,47]. In some patients the benefit is quite dramatic and in others there may be little or no response. A polysomnogram may be considered prior to initiating modafinil to exclude sleep apnea.

What role does rehabilitation play in the treatment of Parkinson's disease? Motor disability in Parkinson's disease may lead to disuse atrophy and contractures. Rehabilitative efforts are often aimed at improving motor function, increasing range of motion, and building endurance. Physical therapy programs generally include therapeutic exercises, gait training, and psychosocial support.

There have been limited evaluations of rehabilitation therapy for Parkinson's disease patients. One open label study identified improvement in strength, initiation of movement, range of motion, and relaxation following a regimen of gymnasium activities [48]. Another study noted improved mobility, feeding, and self care following a home exercise regimen [49]. The most rigorous study to date was a single-blind, randomized, crossover trial evaluating physical disability after four weeks of normal activity and four weeks of intensive physical rehabilitation [50]. Significant improvement in activities of daily living and motor scores were documented following rehabilitation, but scores returned to baseline after six months. Most patients returned to a sedentary lifestyle after structured rehabilitation was completed. This emphasizes the need for long term maintenance physical activity programs.

CHAPTER 9

SURGERY FOR PARKINSON'S DISEASE

What type of surgery is available for patients with Parkinson's disease?

There are three main types of surgery available for patients with PD.1 These include creating a lesion in the brain, deep brain stimulation (DBS) and implantation. Lesion surgeries involve destroying a small target area in the brain. This is usually done by introducing an electrode into the brain with the tip either in the thalamus, globus pallidus or subthalamus. The lesions are usually created by heating the electrode tip for approximately one minute. If the lesion is created in the thalamus the procedure is called **thalamotomy**, in the globus pallidus it is called **pallidotomy** and in the subthalamic nucleus it is called **subthalamotomy.**

An alternative to creating a lesion is stimulation of a target area (Deep Brain Stimulation). A DBS lead with exposed contacts is placed into the target area in the brain. The lead is connected by an extension that runs under the skin to an implantable pulse generator (IPG) placed under the skin, usually below the collar bone. When electrical current is activated it modifies the function of the target site. DBS hardware is manufactured by Medtronic, Inc. There are two kinds of DBS leads available. The intracranial portion of the DBS lead has four contacts which are 1.5 mm in length. One of the leads has contacts separated by 1.5 mm and the second lead has contacts separated by 0.5 mm. There are two kinds of IPGs available, Soletra® and Kinetra® (Not available in the United States). The Kinetra® neurostimulator can be connected to two leads for patients who have undergone DBS procedures on both sides of the brain.

The stimulators can be programmed for monopolar stimulation (one of the four electrodes are turned on) or bipolar (two to four electrodes are turned on) stimulation. Using a hand held computer that is placed over the neurostimulator, the pulse width, amplitude, and stimulation frequency of the electric current generated and the choice of active lead contacts can be adjusted. By using a magnet or Access Review® the patient can turn the device on or off and the Access Review also indicates if the neurostimulator is on or off. The usual stimulation parameters are stimulation frequency of 135 to 185 Hz, pulse width of 60 to 120 microseconds and amplitude of 1 to 3 volts. If the electrode tip is in the thalamus it is called **thalamic stimulation**, in the globus pallidus it is called **pallidal stimulation** and in the subthalamic nucleus it is **subthalamic stimulation.**

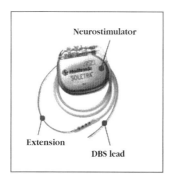

Neurostimulator, Lead and extension, (Medtronic, Inc.)

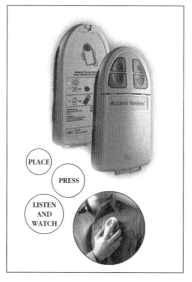

Access Control Device, (Medtronic, Inc.)

Implantation involves delivery of tissue or other material into an area of the brain. It is commonly called transplantation. It is hoped that implanted cells can replace the neurons lost due to the disease and hence restore function. This type of procedure is investigational as the nature of benefit varies depending on the kind of material used for implantation and the benefits observed so far have not been consistent.

Is surgery for Parkinson's disease a new form of therapy?

Surgery for the symptoms of PD has been attempted since the start of the twentieth century.[1] The modern form of surgery using stereotactic procedures was introduced in the 1940s.[2] Stereotactic procedures involve placement of an electrode or probe in the brain using a brain atlas for reference along with neuroimaging for precise targeting. When this from of surgery was initially introduced, the neuroimaging technique that was used was ventriculography. Presently, either computerized tomography (CT) or magnetic resonance imaging (MRI) of the brain are the neuroimaging techniques employed.

Different targets in the brain were explored to find the best area to improve symptoms with the fewest complications. In 1954, lesions were created in the thalamus and this led to the thalamus being considered as the target to control parkinsonian tremor.[3] Stereotactic surgery gained wide recognition and in 1960, Leksell and his team observed that posteroventral pallidotomy helped the major symptoms of PD including tremor, bradykinesia and rigidity.[4] The widespread use of surgery for PD was limited by the associated morbidity and mortality. With the introduction of levodopa in 1967, there was a rapid decline in the use of these procedures until their resurgence in the late 1980s.

Why has there been resurgence in the surgeries for PD?

The limitations in the medical therapy for PD are the major reason for the development of new surgical techniques. When levodopa was initially introduced in 1967 it resulted in marked improvement in symptoms with an associated reduction in morbidity and mortality. However, it was found that with long term use of levodopa patients developed motor fluctuations and dyskinesias and in some patients these symptoms resulted in marked disability. In addition, physicians gained a better understanding of the basal ganglia circuitry and a better understanding of the possible surgical targets for PD. Improved neuroimaging and electrophysiological recording techniques led to greater accuracy of the lesions and resulted in reduced morbidity and mortality associated with these surgeries.

What does the basal ganglia motor circuitry tell us about the possible targets for PD surgery?

The basal ganglia are made up of different nuclei. The main nuclei of the basal ganglia include the caudate, putamen, and globus pallidus and clinicians include the subthalamic nucleus and the substantia nigra. The basal ganglia have connections to the cortex, brain stem nuclei and the thalamus which involve movement. The main pathology in PD is in the substantia nigra which has connections to the striatum (caudate and putamen together are known as the striatum).

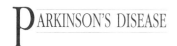

The striatum receives excitatory input from the cortex. In addition, it receives excitatory and inhibitory inputs from the substantia nigra. Striatal output is directed to the medial globus pallidus through two pathways, a direct and indirect pathway. The direct pathway involves inhibitory input to the globus pallidus interna. The indirect pathway involves inhibitory input to the globus pallidus externa which then sends inhibitory input to the subthalamic nucleus which in turn sends excitatory input to the globus pallidus interna. The globus pallidus interna sends inhibitory input to the thalamus which sends excitatory input to the cortex.

In PD, there is loss of substantia nigra neurons and consequently, dopamine in the striatum is reduced. Decreased striatal dopamine diminishes inhibition of the globus pallidus interna (GPi) via the direct pathway and increases stimulation of the GPi via the indirect pathway (figure 1-4). GPi and subthalamic nuclei (STN) are both overactive in PD. There is increased inhibition of the thalamocortical pathway by the GPi which in turn leads to reduced output from the motor cortex. Reduced output from the motor cortex manifests as signs of PD, namely bradykinesia and rigidity.

In PD, a lesion of the GPi would abolish overfiring of the GPi, eliminate the increased inhibition of the thalamocortical pathway and normalize output from the motor cortex (figure 9-1). This could lead to improvement of bradykinesia and rigidity. Similarly, the subthalamic nucleus is also overactive in PD and an STN lesion would reduce overstimulation of the GPi via the indirect pathway (figure 9-2).

Which PD patients are candidates for surgery?

PD patients who have motor fluctuations and dyskinesias that cannot be controlled with medications and patients with disabling tremor that cannot be controlled with medications are candidate for surgery. Patients should not have dementia or other significant medical or behavioral problems. Patients with atypical parkinsonism are not candidates for these surgeries.

Are there any tests to determine if I am a candidate for these procedures?

One needs to undergo evaluation with a neurologist with expertise in surgical therapy. The benefit from surgery is dependent on a correct

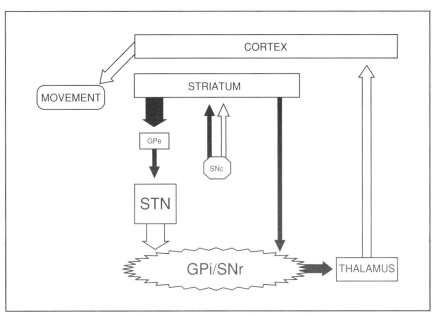

Figure 9-1. *Schematic representation of the effect of pallidotomy. Overfiring of the GPi and resultant excessive inhibition of the thalamocortical pathway are returned toward normal. See text for details.*

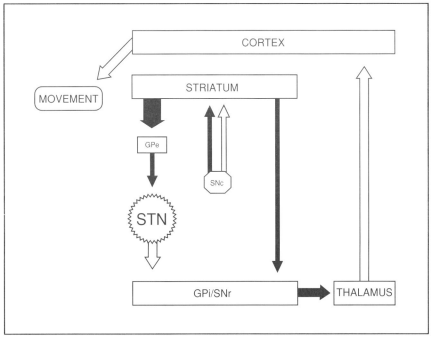

Figure 9-2. *Schematic representation of the effect of subthalamic nucleus lesioning. STN-driven overfiring of the GPi and resultant excessive inhibition of the thalamocortical pathway are returned toward normal.*

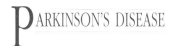

diagnosis of PD. The neurologist will try to determine if the patient has PD or an atypical parkinsonism. Rarely, they may order a positron emission tomography (PET) scan if they have concerns regarding the diagnosis of PD. The neurologist will also determine if symptoms can be improved by further medication adjustments or if surgery is the only option left.

The neurologist will often perform a "levodopa challenge" test to understand the patients response to levodopa. They will evaluate the patient after PD medications are withheld overnight for approximately twelve hours (medication off state) and reevaluate the patient after giving the usual PD medications (medication on state) to determine the extent of the response. This will help predict the possible improvement that can be expected from surgery. MRI of the head is performed to be sure that there are no major strokes or other reasons that surgery should not be performed.

Finally, a memory test, in most cases a complete neuropsychological testing session that takes approximately two to three hours is performed to determine if there are any significant memory problems. These tests will help the neurologist determine if the patient is a possible candidate for surgery. Other routine tests such as blood work and electrocardiogram (EKG) will be performed by the neurosurgeon and the anesthesiologist to be sure that the patient is a surgical candidate and surgery can be safely performed.

How is lesion surgery performed?

On the day of the surgery the patient comes to the hospital, usually without having taken any PD medications. The neurosurgeon usually begins the procedure by attaching a stereotactic frame (a halo-type device) to the patient's head. There are different kinds of frames available. The function of these frames is to stabilize the head during surgery and to help the neurosurgeon determine the precise area to target for surgery. To attach the frame the surgeon uses local anesthesia on four areas around the head. The frame is then attached by four screws to the outer part of the skull. Once the frame is in position, the patient undergoes either a CT of the head or more often, an MRI of the head. The neurosurgeon then uses the brain atlas along with images from the CT or the MRI to determine the exact distances of the target nuclei (thalamus, globus pallidus or the subthalamic nucleus depending on the procedure the patient is about to undergo) and how deep and in what direction the electrode needs to go into the brain. The targeting takes approximately 30 minutes.

After the scan, the patient goes to the operating room (OR). In the OR the patient is put on the operating bed and the head frame is secured to the bed so that the head cannot move but the patient can move other parts of the body. An area on the top of the head is cleaned and shaved. Local anesthesia is injected for the incision. An incision approximately two inches long is made and then a drill is used to make a hole in the skull the size of a nickel. A system to guide the electrode into the brain is then attached to the head frame.

Most neurosurgeons use a technique called microelectrode recording to help locate the precise target area. This technique is used in addition to the initial mapping and targeting. Microelectrode mapping is a technique where a special electrode is passed into the brain. These electrodes detect nearby impulses that are measured and the physicians can estimate the location of the electrode tip depending on the recordings. This process can take approximately two hours.

Once the targeted area is identified, a thermocouple electrode is placed in the brain. Initially the electrode is electrically stimulated to assess for any abnormal sensations or movements, such as muscle spasms. If no abnormal sensations or movements occur, the lesion is created by heating the tip of the electrode for approximately one minute. This destroys the cells at the tip of the electrode. The electrode is removed and the skin incision is sutured and the frame is taken off. General anesthesia is not used for this procedure and the patient is awake through the surgery.

How is deep brain stimulation surgery performed?

The initial procedure is similar to that performed for lesion surgery. Once the target has been localized with the help of microelectrode recordings, the DBS electrode is implanted into the brain. Test stimulation is performed to assess for any abnormal sensations or movements. If there is an appropriate response, the electrode is secured to the skull. If the patient is having bilateral procedures performed, the surgery is repeated on the second side. Once both electrodes are secured to the skull, the incision is sutured and the frame is removed.

The second phase of the surgery is done approximately five to seven days later. This portion is the only part of the surgery that is performed under general anesthesia. An incision is usually made on the top of the head for the extension. The extension is tunneled under the skin of the neck and another incision is made below the collar bone where the stimulator is connected to the extension. The other end of the extension is connected to the DBS lead. Both incisions are sutured and the procedure is repeated on the second side for bilateral procedures.

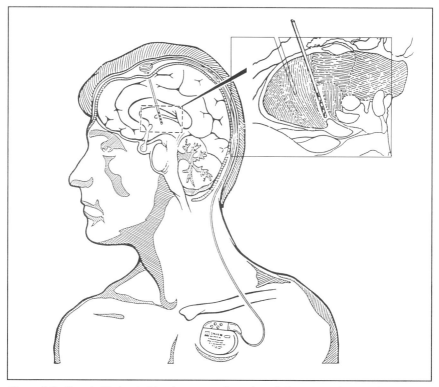

Figure 9-3. *Chronic Thalamic Stimulation. An electrode with four exposed tips is placed into the ventral intermediate (VIM) nucleus of the thalamus. The electrode is attached to a wire which runs beneath the skin to a stimulator placed in the chest wall.*

Are there any contraindications to deep brain stimulation?

DBS is contraindicated in patients who have a medical diagnosis that requires multiple MRI images using full body scan or a head transmit coil that extends to the upper chest. It is also contraindicated in patients in whom test stimulation is unsuccessful and those who do not understand how to use the neurostimulator.

For patients with DBS, diathermy (eg. short wave diathermy, microwave diathermy and therapeutic ultrasound diathermy) is contraindicated because the energy can be transmitted to the brain through the extension and leads and can result in brain tissue damage and possibly death. In addition, diathermy can damage the neurostimulators.

How was the technique of deep brain stimulation developed?

Prior to performing lesions, surgeons use high frequency stimulation to assess improvement in symptoms and any adverse effects before creating the lesion. It was known that patients who undergo bilateral thalamotomy have a relatively high risk of complications, particularly speech and swallowing difficulty. Benabid and colleagues[5] proposed that instead of creating a lesion on the second side in patients who had already undergone thalamotomy, using chronic stimulation could be an option and if patients had significant adverse effects, the stimulation could be reduced or discontinued. Initial studies were promising and hence deep brain stimulation became an option for clinical use.

What are the advantages and disadvantages of DBS over lesion surgery?

The main advantage of DBS surgery is that it is adjustable. The electrical stimulation parameters can be adjusted to improve symptoms or reduced if there are side-effects. In addition, because there is a relatively high risk of bilateral lesion surgery, it is not usually recommended. In contrast, DBS surgery can be performed on both sides with relative safety because the stimulation can be reduced or discontinued if necessary. Another potential advantage is that DBS does not destroy any part of the brain and hence if there are future therapies that can slow the disease progression or cure the disease such therapies could still be used. The disadvantages of DBS surgery include the additional cost of the system and the time and effort involved in programming. Patients may need to undergo repeat surgeries due to device related problems and for battery replacement. The other disadvantage is the risk associated with the use of general anesthesia to implant the stimulator.

What is thalamotomy?

Thalamotomy is a lesion surgery where the probe is introduced into the ventrointermediate (VIM) nucleus of the thalamus and a part of the nucleus is destroyed.

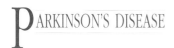

Which patients are candidates for thalamotomy?

Thalamotomy is recommended for patients who have disabling tremor that does not respond to antiparkinsonian medications. These patients should have minimal signs of bradykinesia and rigidity as these symptoms and signs are not improved with thalamotomy. In addition, patients should not have any major memory problems or other unstable medical diagnoses. Patients with a combination of PD tremor and essential tremor are candidates for surgery.

What are the results in patients who have undergone thalamotomy?

Thalamotomies have been performed since the 1950s. However, standardized tests to measure improvements in tremor and other PD signs and symptoms were not initially available. Today, there is improvement in tremor opposite the side of surgery in more than 90% of patients.1 There is a small degree of improvement in rigidity without any improvement in other PD symptoms.

What are the long term benefits of thalamotomy?

There are no well controlled long term studies regarding the efficacy of thalamotomy. Kelly and Gillingham[6] reported their experience in 60 PD patients who underwent thalamotomy between 1965 and 1967. The patients were examined every two years for 10 years. Ninety percent of the 57 patients were free of tremor on the opposite side of the surgery two years later and 57% were still tremor free 10 years after surgery.

Nagaseki and colleagues[7] reported 27 PD patients with a mean follow-up of six and a half years. The beneficial effect of the surgery on tremor was maintained on follow-up. Jankovic and his group[8] reported their results in 42 PD patients with a mean follow-up of approximately 53 months. Eighty six percent of the patients reported moderate to marked improvement of tremor.

Diederich and colleagues[9] reported 17 PD patients with a mean follow-up of approximately 11 years after surgery and noted continued long term benefit for tremor. These studies suggest that there is long term benefit for tremor with thalamotomy.

Why do some patients not experience improvement in tremor with thalamotomy?

Immediately after surgery there is swelling of the brain tissue and this often leads to dramatic improvement of tremor. As the swelling decreases, after a period of two to four weeks, some patients may have recurrence of tremor due to the original lesion not being in the exact location or the lesion being too small. Similarly, some patients can lose benefit long term with thalamotomy as the lesion may become smaller due to scarring. In such patients a repeat thalamotomy or thalamic stimulation may be of benefit.

What is chronic thalamic stimulation?

Chronic thalamic stimulation is an alternative to thalamotomy. The tip of the electrode is left in the ventral intermediate (VIM) nucleus of the thalamus rather than creating a lesion. The electrode is connected to the stimulator as described earlier.

Which patients are candidates for thalamic stimulation surgery?

Patients who are candidates for thalamotomy would also be candidates for thalamic stimulation surgery. In addition, patients who require surgery for both sides of the brain, due to bilateral disabling tremor, would be candidates for this procedure.

What are the benefits of thalamic stimulation?

The majority of studies have reported that tremor is markedly improved with chronic thalamic stimulation. However, this often does not result in improvement in activities of daily living, such as feeding, dressing and tasks involving daily hygiene. Thalamic stimulation does not improve bradykinesia, rigidtiy or drug-induced dyskinesias.

Several studies have evaluated the efficacy of unilateral thalamic stimulation. A 0-4 tremor rating scale is most commonly used where 0 is no tremor and 4 is severe tremor. All studies have reported that the majority of PD patients report improvement in tremor in the contralateral limb.[10-16]

Benabid and colleagues reported 80 PD patients who had thalamic stimulation for medication-resistant tremor.[17] The majority of the patients had

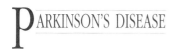

minimal bradykinesia and rigidity. Follow-up done up to 7 years after surgery showed that the tremor continued to be under satisfactory control. There was no dramatic effect on other symptoms including akinesia, rigidity or dyskinesias.

A double-blind multicenter study in 24 PD patients who had undergone unilateral thalamic stimulation reported a significant tremor improvement at one-year, although activities of daily living were not significantly changed.[14] Another multi-center trial with 57 PD patients who had undergone unilateral implant and 16 PD patients who had undergone bilateral implants16 reported tremor was significantly reduced by stimulation. Although symptoms other than tremor were mild, they also reported significant reduction in akinesia and rigidity scores. Another study reported 19 PD patients who demonstrated an 82% reduction in tremor on the side opposite the surgery.[15] However, there was no improvement in activities of daily living or other aspects of PD.

What are the long term benefits of chronic thalamic stimulation?

Lyons and colleagues[18] reported nine PD patients who were followed for an average of 40 months. Although tremor scores continued to be significantly improved patients had worsening of bradykinesia, rigidity and gait due to progression of the disease.

What is pallidotomy?

Pallidotomy is lesion surgery where the probe is introduced into the globus pallidus interna (GPi) and a part of the nucleus is destroyed.

Which patients are candidates for pallidotomy?

Patients with levodopa responsive PD who have disabling symptoms of dyskinesias with motor fluctuations may be candidates for this procedure. Patients should not have significant memory problems. With recent advances in deep brain stimulation, pallidotomy is not usually recommended.

What are the results of pallidotomy?

The majority of studies indicate that pallidotomy is effective for tremor, bradykinesia, and rigidity, and there is marked improvement in the dyskinesias on the side opposite surgery. In a review of 85 articles regarding the efficacy of pallidotomy[19] the results of 1959 PD patients who underwent pallidotomy at 40 centers in 12 countries were reported. The majority of the patients had unilateral pallidotomy. Standardized scales for assessment of improvement in PD symptoms were reported in approximately 25% of the studies at six months and 11% of the studies at one-year. There was basic agreement in these studies that pallidotomy resulted in improvement of motor function in the medication off state and reduced drug induced dyskinesias in the medication on state. At one year, the average improvement in the motor scores in the medication off state was 45% and the reduction in dyskinesias on the side opposite surgery was 86%. There was no consistent improvement in motor symptoms in the medication on state.

What are the long term benefits of pallidotomy?

Lang and colleagues[20] reported 11 PD patients two years after pallidotomy and reported that the improvement in off state motor scores and on state dyskinesias was sustained. However, the initial improvements in balance and gait were lost after six months. Another study reported that although unilateral pallidotomy was useful in controlling dyskinesias and tremor three years after surgery, all other benefits disappeared and activities of daily living continued to worsen.[21] Hariz and colleagues[22] reported the course of 13 PD patients approximately 10 years after pallidotomy. Five patients required additional surgery for their PD symptoms. Dosages of antiparkinsonian medications were increased in all patients without any increase in dyskinesias on the side opposite surgery. There was progression of bradykinesia, worsening of gait and eventual decline in cognition.

What is globus pallidus interna (GPi) stimulation?

GPi stimulation is an alternative to pallidotomy. The tip of the electrode is left in the globus pallidus interna rather than creating a lesion. The electrode is connected to the stimulator as described earlier.

What patients are candidates for GPi stimulation?

Patients with levodopa responsive PD who have disabling symptoms of dyskinesias with motor fluctuations may be candidates for the procedure. Patients should not have significant memory problems. Patients usually require electrodes on both sides.

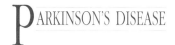

What are the results of GPi stimulation?

Similar to pallidotomy, the most consistent effect of GPi stimulation is a marked reduction of levodopa induced dyskinesias. The improvement in parkinsonian symptoms in the medication off state has been reported to be 27-50%.[23-26] Improvement in activities of daily living has ranged from 19% to 68%. Improvement in on medication scores has not been consistent and in fact some investigators have reported a worsening. All studies reported a significant reduction in dyskinesias resulting in an increase in on time during the day.

Most of the studies of GPi stimulation have evaluated small series of patients. A multicenter study of bilateral GPi stimulation reported results from multiple countries.[24] Forty-one patients were enrolled and electrodes were implanted in 38 patients (two patients had cerebral hemorrhage and one patient had intraoperative confusion). In the off-medication state, all of the cardinal features of PD improved. Tremor scores improved by 59%, rigidity improved by 31%, bradykinesia improved by 26%, gait by 35% and postural instability by 36%. Patient diaries revealed that the percentage of on time without dyskinesias during awake time increased from 28 to 64% and off time was reduced from 37 to 24%. The mean dose of antiparkinsonian medications was unchanged between baseline and six months.

What are the long term benefits of GPi stimulation?

Long term follow-up results of GPi stimulation are lacking. Ghika et al[25] reported six PD patients with a minimum follow-up of 24 months. Although improvements persisted beyond two years after surgery, signs of decreased efficacy were seen after 12 months. Another report evaluated six patients for approximately three years.[27] Dyskinesia severity and activities of daily living continued to be significantly improved. However, improvement in mean daily duration of off time was lost at the last assessment.

What is subthalamic nucleus (STN) stimulation?

The STN is a small nucleus, approximately the size of a bean (7mm x 9mm x 5mm).[28] STN stimulation is when the electrode tip is in the STN nucleus. Similar to thalamic and GPi stimulation the electrodes are connected to stimulators.

Which patients are candidates for STN stimulation?

Patients with levodopa responsive PD who have motor fluctuations and dyskinesias that cannot be improved by medication adjustments are candidates for this procedure. Patients should not have memory problems or behavioral problems such as severe depression.

What are the results of STN stimulation?

There are multiple reports of the antiparkinsonian effects of STN stimulation.[24, 29-31] Reports have noted improvements in all motor symptoms of PD including tremor, rigidity, bradykinesia, posture and gait in the medication off state. There is marked improvement in dyskinesias due to reduction in antiparkinsonian medications after surgery and improvement in the duration of on time. Improvement in activities of daily living has ranged from 30-72% and motor score improvements have ranged from 42-74% in the off-medication state. Antiparkinsonian medications are usually reduced by 37-80% after surgery resulting in a 63-81% reduction in dykinesias.

One of the largest studies of STN stimulation is a multicenter study that was performed in multiple countries.[24] Ninety-six patients had bilateral STN implants. In the off-medication state there was a mean improvement of 44% in activities of daily living and a mean improvement of 51% in motor scores. All motor subscores in the off-medication state also improved; tremor scores by 79%, rigidity by 58%, bradykinesia by 42%, gait by 56% and postural instability by 50%. Patient home diaries revealed the off-state during the day decreased by 61%, on-state improved by 174% [CHECK] and on-state with dyskinesias decreased by 70%. Although there was some improvement in the on-state scores it was not as robust.

What are the long term results for STN stimulation surgery?
Long term studies of STN stimulation surgery are limited. Benabid et al[32] have followed more than 50 patients for one year, 30 patients for two years, 16 patients for three years, nine patients for four years and four patients for five years. These patients have observed adequate control of the motor features of PD and reductions in levodopa dose have persisted. A tendency towards increased speech difficulties and midline motor features such as gait and balance difficulties has been observed. Rodriquez et al[33] reported results in nine patients between 30 and 36 months after

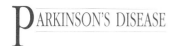

surgery and the patients continued to have a 61% reduction in motor scores and a 38% reduction in levodopa dosage.

What is subthalamotomy?

Subthalamotomy refers to creating a lesion in the STN. Subthalamotomy is not usually recommended in United States. However, due to the cost of deep brain stimulation hardware there is interest in this procedure, especially in less developed countries. Different series have reported that the results are similar to STN stimulation, however risks of dyskinesias and intracranial complications appear to be higher than with stimulation.[34]

Is bilateral STN stimulation surgery superior to bilateral GPi surgery? Although the criteria for patient selection for GPi and STN targets are similar, there are no large studies that have randomly compared these two procedures. Krack et al[31] compared eight patients who underwent STN stimulation and five patients who underwent GPi. In the off-state, the there was a 71% improvement in the PD symptoms with STN stimulation and a 39% improvement with GPi stimulation. Rigidity and tremor showed good improvement in both groups but bradykinesia was more improved in the STN group. There was a reduction in levodopa dosage only in the STN group.

Burchiel et al[35] performed a randomized study in 10 PD patients with five patients undergoing GPi and five STN stimulation. At 12 months there was a similar improvement in both groups. However, only patients who underwent STN stimulation had a reduction in antiparkinsonian medications.

Volkmann et al[36] reported a 54% improvement in parkinsonian signs with GPi stimulation as compared to a 67% improvement with STN. Medication was reduced only in the STN group. These and other studies show a greater improvement in patients who have undergone STN stimulation as compared to GPi stimulation. Therefore, most surgery centers favor STN stimulation over GPi stimulation.

What are the side-effects of deep brain stimulation surgery?

Side-effects of deep brain stimulation surgery are relatively similar for the three targets (thalamic, GPi and STN) and can be divided into those related to the surgical procedure, those associated with the device and those associated with stimulation. These complications are to some extent dependent on the expertise of the neurosurgeon, the proper patient selection and the mechanical problems associated with the equipment.

Surgical Complications

Surgical complications usually occur within 30 days of surgery. These complications are similar to those that occur with other forms of brain surgery and usually occur in less than 5% of patients. These complications include intracranial bleeds, strokes, seizures and infections. Rare cases of death have also been reported. Pollack et al[37] assessed 212 patients who had undergone thalamic, GPi or STN stimulation and reported two deaths. One death was due to pulmonary embolism and another occurred three years after surgery in a patient who had an intracranial bleed. In this series, permanent complications occurred in seven patients (2.3%); three had intracerebral bleeds, three patients developed dementia and one patient had an unrelated traumatic hematoma. Other transient events include seizures, post operative confusion, bleeding under the skin, speech difficulty, numbness, weakness and other nerve injuries. The majority of these events resolve within 30 days.

Hardware related

Initial misplacement of the lead may require repeat surgery to correct the exact lead tip position. Other potential problems include displacement of the electrode, erosion of the skin over the lead or the extension, breakage of the lead or malfunction of the electrical system, including the stimulator. These device-related events can occur in up to 25% of the patients.[38] Oh et al[38] reported 79 patients who had 124 leads implanted as some of them were on both sides. Twenty patients had some form of hardware related problems. These included four lead breaks, movement of four leads, three electrical problems, 12 skin erosions or infections, and two reactions due to the presence of hardware in the body. Pollack et al[37] in their series of 300 patients reported that infection or skin erosion occurred in 10 patients, breakage of lead connection in seven patients and stimulator repositioning in five patients.

Stimulation Related

Side-effects related to stimulation depend on the exact location of the tip of the lead and the intensity of stimulation. The majority of these side-effects can be reduced by either using another lead contact or by reducing the stimulation intensity. These side-effects include eye lid closure, double vision, muscle spasms, tingling, numbness, speech difficulties, depression,

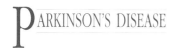

mood changes, increased sexual desires, vision changes, balance difficulties, and pain. Occasionally nonspecific sensations such as anxiety, panic, palpitations, nausea and strange sensations can also occur. In some patients reducing the stimulation intensity or changing the lead contact may reduce the side-effects but may also lead to loss of benefit. In some patients, additional surgery may be required to change the location of the lead. Depression, manic behavior, increased sexual desire, balance difficulties and speech difficulties can be very bothersome, and some patients may require medications to control these side-effects.

How does deep brain stimulation surgery work?

The exact way that deep brain stimulation works is unknown. As the benefits of deep brain stimulation are similar to those observed after creating lesions in the thalamus, GPi and STN it was believed that deep brain stimulation works by reducing the overactivity in these nuclei. The other possibility is that the electrical discharges from these nuclei become abnormal and irregular in patients with PD. Deep brain stimulation resets the electrical discharges and makes them regular.

What is the concept behind transplantation as a surgical treatment for Parkinson's disease?

The basic idea of transplantation is to replace lost dopamine neurons.

Why is Parkinson's disease an attractive target for transplantation?

Parkinson's disease is an attractive target disease for transplantation because the degeneration is relatively site and neuron specific (dopamine neurons of the nigrostriatal pathway), the striatal implantation area is relatively large, and clinical benefit can be attained with neurotransmitter replacement rather than being dependent on restoration of neuronal circuitry.

What cells were considered candidates for transplantation?

Fetal human dopamine cells were considered as candidates for transplantation because these cells normally grow and connect with the correct target neurons. It was hoped that this property of fetal cells would allow them to replace neurons lost to the disease process.

Do animal studies indicate that fetal cell transplantation is a viable procedure?

Studies in animal models of Parkinson's disease have demonstrated that transplanted fetal mesencephalic neurons survive, form synaptic connections, exhibit normal firing patterns, and improve parkinsonian features [39-50]. These studies also indicate that implantation of appropriate tissue into an appropriate location is necessary for clinical benefit.

What was the first transplantation strategy employed in Parkinson's disease?

Autologous adrenal medullary transplantation was the first transplant strategy used in Parkinson's disease because it was not encumbered by the logistic, ethical and immunologic issues surrounding fetal cell transplantation. In animal studies, adrenal cell transplantation was found to provide some benefit although this was limited and not as great as was observed using fetal tissue.

What were the results of adrenal transplantation in Parkinson's disease patients?

The first attempts at adrenal transplantation began in 1982 and were found to bring about only minimal and transient improvement [51,52]. However, in 1987, Madrazo and coworkers reported "dramatic amelioration" of symptoms in two young patients [53].

Subsequent investigators noted only modest improvement in function during OFF time and a mild reduction of OFF time [54-63]. Most of this benefit was lost by two years [64]. Patients who came to autopsy were found to have few or no surviving transplanted cells [58,65-68]. This procedure has now been abandoned.

What were the results of the first attempts at fetal cell grafting in Parkinson's disease?

Lindvall and coworkers first evaluated fetal grafting in two patients using a mesencephalic cell suspension from single donors [69,70]. These patients experienced modest but significant improvement in motor function while OFF. Two additional patients received cell suspension grafts from four donors [71,72]. These patients experienced gradual improvement beginning six to 12 weeks after surgery. Motor function

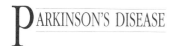

while OFF progressively improved and OFF time decreased. Improvement in bradykinesia and rigidity was observed bilaterally but was most pronounced on the contralateral side.

Fluorodopa PET studies demonstrated improved dopaminergic function beginning one year after transplant[73]. This experience indicated that clinical improvement might be dependent on transplanting a sufficient amount of tissue. Several other groups have also reported modest benefit with transplant using a single donor[74-76].

In contrast, more benefit was observed in two patients with MPTP-induced parkinsonism[77]. These patients received bilateral transplants using tissue from three to four donors per side. It is possible that greater improvement occurred because these patients had MPTP-induced parkinsonism rather than Parkinson's disease. Alternatively, they may have experienced more benefit due to the greater amount of tissue transplanted.

What were the results of early fetal cell transplantation studies?

Several hundred PD patients received transplanted human mesencephalic tissue, mostly in small, unblinded trials at multiple investigational sites[78-95]. Transplanted patients were mostly those with disability related to motor fluctuations that could not be overcome with additional medication manipulation[96]. Fetal transplants were prepared as blocks of tissue or suspensions of dissociated cells. Donor age varied from 5 to 17 weeks post-conception, and 3 to 5 fetal nigra were generally transplanted per side into the striatum. Some studies employed immunosuppression while others did not. Many of these studies found that transplanted dopamine neurons survived transplantation, and led to clinical motor improvement over several months to years, with reductions in OFF time, improvement in UPDRS scores, decreased dyskinesia, and lowering of levodopa doses. One study found 32% improvement in UPDRS total OFF scores 20 months following transplantation in 6 patients[91]. ON time without dyskinesia improved from 22 to 60% and FD uptake was significantly increased at 6 (48%) and 12 months (61%). Increases in FD uptake were correlated with clinical improvement on UPDRS scoring. Two subjects died 18 months after surgery from unrelated causes and autopsies demonstrated healthy appearing transplanted cells numbering 82,000 to 138,000 per side[87].

Another study found that in 6 transplanted patients evaluated at one year and four patients evaluated at two years, OFF UPDRS scores were improved 18 and 26% and OFF time was reduced 34 and 44%. FD uptake increased 68% at 8-12 months[92].

Autopsies performed on two transplanted patients demonstrated healthy graft tissue, including large numbers of surviving dopaminergic cells and physiologic reinnervation patterns[80,87]. Transplanted grafts extended neuritic process 2 to 7 mm[96]. Grafting at 5 mm intervals resulted in reinnervation of up to 78% of the postcommissural putamen, and survival of dopamine neurons following grafting ranged from 5% to 20%. No graft rejection was observed, although immune markers were activated[97].

PET scans following transplantation in many open label studies demonstrated increased fluorodopa uptake in the graft area[78,87,96,98], consistent with graft survival. Piccini et al. demonstrated synaptic dopamine release from embryonic nigral transplants using raclopride positron emission tomography in a patient who had received a transplant in the right putamen 10 years earlier, and experienced sustained, marked clinical benefit[93].

Thus, evidence from open label studies indicated that transplanted embryonic mesencephalic cells could survive transplantation, uptake DOPA as seen on PET scans, at least partially reinnervate the striatum, and release dopamine into the synapse. In addition, these studies suggested clinical benefit, especially with regard to improving motor function during the OFF state and decreasing OFF time. However, any clinical benefit observed in open label studies could potentially be due in part or whole to placebo effects. A reliable evaluation of the clinical benefits of fetal cell transplantation required double blind, sham surgery-controlled studies[99].

What were the results of fetal cell transplantation in double-blind studies?

Freed et al. evaluated transplantation of embryonic dopamine neurons into 40 advanced PD patients in a double-blind, sham surgery-controlled trial[100]. Patients (34 to 75 years of age, mean disease duration 14 years) were randomly assigned to undergo transplantation or sham surgery, and were followed in a double-blind manner for one year, after which time those in the sham surgery group were offered transplantation.

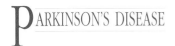

Mesencephalic tissue from a total of four embryos was transplanted into the putamen bilaterally. All patients had PD for more than seven years, and had previously responded favorably to levodopa.

The primary outcome measure was a subjective global rating of the change in the disease that was mailed in by patients 12 months following surgery. The global rating was scored on a scale of −3 to +3, corresponding to phrases including "parkinsonism markedly worse (-3)", to "parkinsonism markedly improved (+3)" compared to baseline. According to this scale, there was not a significant difference between transplanted and non-transplanted groups. The mean (± SD) global rating score was 0.0 ± 2.1 for transplanted patients compared to −0.4 ± 1.7 for sham surgery patients (p=0.62).

Total UPDRS OFF scores were not different across groups at one year. However, younger patients who were transplanted had a 28% improvement in total UPDRS scores (p = 0.01) compared to the sham-surgery group. UPDRS OFF motor scores decreased 18% for the whole transplantation group (p = 0.04), and 34% for the younger patients (P = 0.005). 18F-fluorodopa uptake in the putamen on positron emission tomography increased 40 ± 42% in the transplanted group compared to a decline of 2 ± 17% in the sham-surgery group (p=0.001). Autopsy results in two patients who died from causes unrelated to surgery revealed 2,000 to 23,000 surviving transplanted dopamine neurons per transplant track.

Thus, although the change in the global rating scale was not significantly different between groups, various secondary outcome variables suggest that there was some clinical benefit, especially for the younger patients. Nonetheless, the lack of difference in the global rating scale suggests that any benefits observed were not sufficient to meaningfully impact overall function in these patients.

Were there any major side-effects from fetal cell transplantation?

Thirty-three patients in this study ultimately received transplants and were followed for as long as three years after surgery. Dystonia and dyskinesia that persisted after elimination or reduction of antiparkinsonian therapy ("runaway dyskinesias") occurred in five (15%) of the 33 patients more than one year after surgery. The cause of these dyskinesias despite discontinuation of medication is poorly understood, but to some extent appears to be related to unregulated dopamine release from grafts [101].

Have there been other double-blind studies of human fetal transplantation?

In another study, thirty-four advanced PD patients were randomized to receive bilateral transplantation with one donor per side, four donors per side, or sham procedures [102].

Patients were followed for two years and the primary outcome variable was UPDRS motor score during "practically defined OFF" (in the morning after medication had been withheld for at least 12 hours. Thirty-one patients completed the trial, and two died during the trial and three afterward, all for causes unrelated to the surgery. Patients who received transplantation with four donors demonstrated very well innervated striata on autopsy. PET results demonstrated a significant dose-dependent increase in fluorodopa uptake with no change in sham-surgery patients and an approximate one-third increase in patients receiving four donors.

No significant differences were identified in clinical measures following transplantation. Increases (worsening) compared to baseline in UPDRS motor scores while off medication were 9.4 for placebo, 3.5 for one donor and -0.72 for four donors (p=0.096 for 4 vs placebo). Transplanted patients improved for approximately 9 months, possibly suggesting a delayed immune response. Thirteen of 23 transplanted patients developed off-medication dyskinesias and three required surgical treatment to control them. No off-medication dyskinesia was observed in sham-surgery patients.

How would you summarize the results of these studies?

Double-blind studies thus confirm that transplanted fetal mesencephalic cells can survive transplantation as evidenced by both autopsy studies and increased FD uptake. These studies have not demonstrated definitive benefit, although they do suggest modest clinical benefit in various measures of parkinsonian severity. Further study is required to determine why such limited clinical benefit is achieved relative to cell survival and apparent striatal reinnervation.

Evaluation of graft dopamine release and postsynaptic stimulation on a microanatomic level may be necessary. The development of off-medication dyskinesia has been identified as a significant adverse event in a substantial proportion of transplanted patients. This represents a critical hurdle that must be overcome if transplantation is to be developed into a useful clinical therapy. Further study is required to learn the basis of off-medication dyskinesia to understand how they might be avoided.

What were the results of transplantation of porcine (pig) dopamine cell transplantation?

Although an open label study suggested possible clinical benefit (103,104), a subsequent double-blind study did not identify significant improvement comparing transplanted to imitation surgery patients [105]. Transplanted patients demonstrated a mean improvement in total UPDRS score in the OFF state at 18 months of 24.6 ± 25.0% and non-transplanted patients demonstrated a mean improvement of 21.6 ± 14.0% ($p = 0.6$).

This experience highlights the fact that substantial placebo effect can be seen in surgical trials in PD and points up the need for definitive randomized double-blind sham-surgery controlled studies.

What is the status of human retinal cell transplantation?

Transplanted cultured human retinal pigment epithelial cells (RPE) are currently being evaluated as a source of dopamine dopa that may improve parkinsonian symptoms. RPE cells are harvested from the posterior layer of the retina next to the choroid [106], and have been shown to survive in rodent and non-human primate models with minimal host immune response while improving parkinsonian symptoms.

Watts et al. evaluated the safety and efficacy of unilateral RPE transplantation in 6 advanced PD patients in an open-label pilot study [107]. RPE cells attached to cross-linked gelatin microcarriers (Spheramine) were implanted into the post-commissural putamen contralateral to the worst affected side and no immunosuppression was used. At six and nine months following surgery, motor UPDRS scores improved 33% and 42%, respectively from preoperative baseline scores in six patients. Double-blind studies are now underway to provide a definitive evaluation.

What is the status of stem cell transplantation?

The field of stem cell biology is still in its infancy and many hurdles remain to be overcome. The hope is that stem cells will provide an unlimited, self-renewing source of cells that can be transplanted, migrate to areas of injury or degeneration, and replace lost cells by differentiating into the appropriate cell type and integrating into host neuronal circuitry.

It has been surprisingly difficult to achieve a complete and coordinated induction of multipotent stem cells into a single cell type. In the laboratory, stem cells are exposed to a variety of complex manipulations and exposures to growth factors and other signals to induce differentiation into dopamine neurons[108]. However, to date most of these regimens are plagued by a relatively low proportion of resultant dopamine cells or a poor cell survival rate following grafting. It seems likely, though, that further refinements to the differentiation and maintenance regimens will improve this situation over time.

What other surgical approaches are being developed?

An alternative approach is the delivery of neurotrophic factors. At this time, most interest is focused on the delivery of glial derived neurotrophic factor (GDNF). Potential methods of delivery include viral gene transfer, direct infusion, and stem cell delivery. Viral delivery of GDNF in aged monkeys has been demonstrated to increase the number of dopamine neurons and protect against MPTP toxicity[109]. GDNF-producing stem cells prevented the degeneration of dopamine neurons in mice after intrastriatal injection of 6-OHDA and reduced amphetamine and apomorphine induced turning[110].

Can GDNF be infused directly into the brain?

A small open label pilot study of continuous direct infusion of GDNF in PD patients has shown promise[111]. Improvement was observed in all five patients who underwent the infusion. In the practically defined OFF state (in the morning, off all antiparkinsonian medications at least 12 hours) ADL, motor, and total Unified Parkinson's Disease Rating scale (UPDRS) scores and time motor tests improved. It is estimated that mean total UPDRS OFF scores and OFF timed motor tests improved approximately 50%. In addition, ON time through the day increased, OFF time decreased, and dyskinesia severity and duration decreased. Side-effects were limited. Double-blind studies are required to accurately assess the potential benefit of GDNF infusion.

CHAPTER 10

QUESTIONS FREQUENTLY ASKED BY PATIENTS

Is exercise important for patients with Parkinson's disease?

Exercise is extremely important in Parkinson's disease. Exercise helps maintain the best possible function in the face of a progressive disorder. The saying, "Use it or lose it" applies. For example, a walking regimen helps maintain the ability to walk. In addition, exercise provides the added benefits of improving mood, energy level, and sleep.

Have studies demonstrated that exercise is beneficial?

Yes, exercise programs have been shown to produce improvement in gait, grip strength, and motor coordination [1]. In one study, a 13-week exercise program consisting of supervised and unsupervised home exercises was associated with significant improvement in gait [2]. Another study demonstrated improvement in range of motion as a result of an exercise program consisting of climbing stairs, hitting a punching bag, and catching a ball [3].

What types of exercises are important?

Exercises for mobility, stretching, and strengthening are all important. Mobility exercises help maintain walking ability. A stretching regimen improves flexibility and helps fight the tendency for stooped posture. Increased strength will help maintain mobility and function even as slowness and stiffness progress.

How often should I exercise?

At least three or four times per week, and preferably every day. The amount of time spent exercising each day is partly a function of tolerance, but most patients should exercise for at least twenty minutes per session.

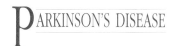

If you cannot tolerate twenty minutes at a time, divide it up through the day, and try to build up your tolerance. Patients with early disease can usually tolerate 40 minutes to an hour of exercise per session.

Doesn't the exercise regimen depend on the stage of the disease?

Yes, the type of exercise that's right for a particular person depends on functional ability. A young person with early disease may play tennis, swim laps, jog, or ride a bicycle. For patients who are a little older or who have a little more advanced disease, exercise activities might include golf, light swimming, walking in a pool, or using a stationary bicycle or rowing machine. For patients with moderate disease, a walking regimen is very important. During hot or cold weather, many patients like to walk indoors. A shopping mall is often a good place to walk because it is temperature-controlled and the floor is usually flat and not slippery. Walkers can be used in a mall if necessary. For patients who are unable to walk, mobility, stretching and strengthening exercises that can be done in a chair are appropriate.

It is important to find physical activities that you like to do so that you will continue them over time. A long term program is necessary because studies have shown that the benefit of exercise is lost when patients discontinue their regimen [4]. Engage in physical activity that is at the right level for you. Activities that create undue risk should be avoided. The importance of moderate exercise cannot be stressed enough and it is not believed that overdoing it, such as training for a marathon, is either necessary or helpful.

Are rehabilitation programs helpful?

Rehabilitation programs can help tailor a regimen to suit your needs. A physical therapist will evaluate your function, abilities, and limitations and will design a program based on that evaluation. In addition, rehabilitation programs give you a "jump start", to get you going on your exercise program. However, you must keep up the program once you have completed rehabilitation to maintain the benefit. Be sure to receive clear instructions as to what regimen is recommended once you have completed the initial program.

If you are considering a rehabilitation program, it is recommended that you meet with the personnel to discuss what services will be provided. You will also want to know the cost, and what may be covered by insurance.

What types of therapists make up a rehabilitation program?

Physical therapists perform a functional evaluation, design a physical rehabilitation program, and assist you in carrying out the program. They might also recommend assistive devices for ambulating such as a walker. Occupational therapists perform a functional evaluation concentrating on fine finger and hand movements. They recommend exercises and adaptive devices to improve hand and arm function.

Occupational therapists also perform home evaluations to determine if modifications would be helpful. They might determine that handrails are needed in the shower to help prevent falls or that a trapeze device would help you to get out of bed or turn over at night. Speech therapists evaluate voice amplitude and clarity. They often provide speech exercises and teach patients techniques to help them communicate better.

Speech therapists also evaluate swallowing. Swallowing is assessed by observation and in some cases a special test called a barium swallow will be needed. Based on the swallowing evaluation, a speech therapist will make recommendations regarding optimal food texture and thickening liquids, and teach techniques to make swallowing easier and safer.

I have Parkinson's disease and am having trouble with balance. My physician recommends that I get a walking device. Which one should I purchase?

Wheeled walkers may prevent falls in patients with balance difficulty and can improve mobility [5]. Two, three, and four-wheeled walkers are available. The 3-wheeled walker is shaped like a triangle. One study compared 2- and 3-wheeled walkers and found the 3-legged, 3-wheeled models preferable. Subjects walked faster and had greater maneuverability with the 3-wheeled walker [5]. We prefer the 3-legged, 3-wheeled walker with hand brakes for patients who are able to use it.

Before purchasing a walking device, visit a medical supply store and try out different varieties. Determine which one works best for you.

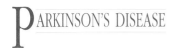

I have Parkinson's disease and I am speaking too softly. What can I do to improve this?

Approximately 60 to 90% of PD patients exhibit speech or voice abnormalities [6] including reduced volume, diminished articulation, decreased variation in tone, tremor [7], or hoarseness [8]. Patients may lose clarity of speech and articulation of consonants is less precise. Particularly difficult are the sounds of the letters k,g,f,v,s, and z [9]. Just as there may be decreased dexterity in fine finger movements, there is also a loss of dexterity in the muscles involved in articulation. Decreased control and strength of airflow, and rigidity of the laryngeal muscles may also contribute to speech difficulty [8].

In some patients there is bowing of the vocal cords so that they do not lie in contact with each other to capture airflow and vibrate. For these patients, collagen injections into the vocal cords may remarkably improve speech [10]. ENT specialists perform this procedure as well as a specialized evaluation to assess whether the procedure might offer benefit. Increasing antiparkinsonian mediation may improve speech but there are often limitations as to how much benefit can be achieved with medication adjustments alone [11]. Voice rehabilitation is beneficial in improving vocal intensity and articulation [12]. Ask your physician to refer you to a speech therapist for exercises you can perform at home.

How can I maximize the benefit of my visit to the doctor?

Recognize that the time the doctor can spend with you is limited. The better prepared you are, the more time your doctor will have to address your questions and concerns. Bring a list of *all* your medications, the doses, and the times you take them. It may be helpful to bring your medications in their labeled containers in case questions arise.

You should tell the doctor what aspect of your Parkinson's disease is currently causing you the most difficulty. You may also want to discuss the next one or two biggest problems. We suggest that you determine in advance what three problems you most want to discuss. It is usually not possible to address more than three problems at a single visit. You might mention more than three if they are important to you, but focus on three or less to be addressed and discussed.

If something is on your mind, particularly medication changes that you think might be beneficial, be sure to bring it up for consideration. If the doctor suggests changes that you do not think will be helpful, be sure to tell him so that he will have a chance to discuss it further or reconsider his recommendations.

I have motor fluctuations and dyskinesia. What additional information will my doctor want?

If you are experiencing motor fluctuations, your doctor will want to know how long it takes for your levodopa to start to work, and how long the benefit lasts. He will want to know how much of the day, while you are awake, the medication is providing benefit ("on" time) and how much of the day you are not experiencing benefit because the medication has worn off ("off" time).

If you are having dyskinesia (twisting, turning movements) he will want to know how much of the day they are present, and how troublesome they are, if at all. He will also want to know what causes you more difficulty, "off" time or dyskinesia.

I don't like anyone else in the room with me during my doctor's visit. Is that OK?

We strongly believe that someone else should be in the room with you during your office visit, preferably a spouse or caregiver. It is often valuable for the doctor to get additional information from a second person who knows how you are doing at home. Another perspective may help emphasize certain problems. In addition, your spouse or caregiver may have their own questions or concerns that need to be addressed. It is helpful when two people listen to the discussion in case one forgets after the visit is over.

What should I take with me when I leave the doctor's office?

You should receive written instructions detailing any medication changes and these should be clear to you before you leave the office. If the instructions are not clear, ask for additional clarification. You may want to refer to the written instructions at home in case you can't remember or if uncertainty arises later. A copy of your written instructions should be placed in your medical chart so that this is available if you call with questions or a problem occurs.

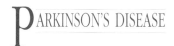

How often should I see my doctor for my Parkinson's disease?

Patients who are stable and doing reasonably well might be seen about every four months. This usually provides the opportunity to make medication changes before there has been too much progression in symptoms. Most patients should be seen no less frequently than every six months. If visits are less often than six months, disease progression without medication adjustment may cause unnecessary discomfort and disability. Patients are seen more frequently than every four months if multiple medication adjustments are required so as not to waste time. If a new medication is introduced that needs to be monitored, or if further adjustments are expected, the next visit is scheduled sooner.

My doctor gave me a prescription for a new medication. I bought a months supply only to find I could not tolerate the medication. How can I avoid this happening in the future?

When a new medication is prescribed, ask your doctor if samples are available to see if you can tolerate it before buying more. You can also ask you pharmacist to initially dispense a few days supply before filling the rest of the prescription.

My medication is very expensive and my insurance plan does not cover it. Can I get help with the cost of my medication?

If the cost of medication is an issue be sure to let your doctor know. He can then consider cost more strongly when he formulates a treatment plan. Some medications are more expensive than others.

Ask your doctor about generic medications. In most cases, if a generic formulation is available it will be less expensive than the name brand. Remember that a generic does not always contain exactly the same amount of medication as the name brand even if the pill is the same "dose". Patients who are sensitive to small changes in dose may prefer the name brand.

Most pharmaceutical companies have programs to provide medication for patients who are truly unable to afford it. An application that includes your financial information should be submitted to the company to see if you qualify for the program. Ask your physician for the name, address, and phone number of the company that distributes the medication, and contact the company.

My physician has diagnosed me with Parkinson's disease, but I would like a second opinion. Where should I go to get one?

Contact one of the information and referral sources listed at the end of this chapter. They will provide the name of a Movement Disorder or Parkinson's disease specialist, who will be happy to provide a second opinion. Do not be afraid or embarrassed to obtain a second opinion, and bring all scans and records with you.

Should I join a support group?

Support groups are very valuable. They are a tremendous source of information regarding the disease, coping mechanisms, treatment options, local doctors, and support services. They provide a sense of community and shared experience. Support groups serve as a forum to express frustrations and to share your knowledge.

I am scheduled to undergo surgery for another medical problem. Is there anything special I need to know?

Because of possible serious complications due to the interaction of selegiline and anesthesia or narcotics, selegiline should be discontinued at least ten days prior to elective surgery.

You should discuss with your doctors how you should handle your other antiparkinsonian medications. In order to avoid worsening mobility, breathing, and swallowing that may occur if patients are off medications for more than a few hours, antiparkinsonian medications should usually be taken right up to the time of surgery and reinstituted as soon after surgery as possible. Immediately after surgery your stomach and intestine may not be functioning and absorbing medications normally, and you may find that even though you are taking your medications you may not get a response.

While in the hospital, patients with confusion or hallucinations may experience a worsening of these symptoms due to the unfamiliar environment. Pain medications, sedatives, and infections can also worsen confusion and hallucinations.

Because of these potential problems, it is recommended that patients with advanced PD have their surgery at a hospital where a neurologist who is familiar with them and knowledgeable about PD is available to provide care.

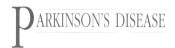

Am I at increased risk for complications from surgery because of my disease?

Patients with more advanced disease have a higher complication rate following surgery. One study found that the average length of hospital stay was more than two days longer for Parkinson's disease patients than non-parkinsonian patients [13]. Parkinson's disease patients had more urinary tract infections, pneumonia, and other bacterial infections. This higher complication rate probably reflects diminished mobility, breathing, and swallowing [14]. Patients who are immobile may have urinary catheters in place longer, thereby causing urinary tract infections [13]. It is important to have catheters and other lines taken out as soon as they are no longer needed and to be out of bed as soon and as often as is feasible.

In considering whether you should have a particular operation, you and your doctor should weigh the relative benefits and risks in light of this higher complication rate.

My husband has Parkinson's disease and I am concerned about his driving. What should I do?

Driving requires high level motor and thinking skills, good judgment, and quick reaction times. Advanced PD and cognitive impairment are associated with higher accident rates [15]. Unfortunately, the patient is often unaware of diminished driving ability and it usually falls on the spouse or other family members to detect driving problems. This can cause conflict within a family, as some patients are unwilling to stop driving even when told it is unsafe. A driving simulator test can provide an objective assessment of driving ability, or the patient can be referred to a motor vehicle agency for a driving evaluation. If you have concerns about your spouse's driving ability, let your physician know. Although sympathetic to the loss of independence that comes with loss of driving ability, patient safety and the safety of everyone on the road is the paramount consideration.

I am 57 years old and I am having difficulty doing my job. I have just been diagnosed with Parkinson's disease. Should I continue working or should I consider disability or early retirement?

Avoid a hasty decision. Treatment may improve your symptoms such that you may be able to do your job without much difficulty. It is usually wise to gauge your response to medication before making any long term employment decisions. If you feel your job is threatened because of poor performance, it is important to convey this to your doctor.

Approximately thirty to forty percent of PD patients stop working early[16,17]. However, lost wages and earnings are a potential family burden and source of stress[18]. You will want to carefully weigh the pros and cons of retiring early. An important consideration is medical insurance. Unless special arrangements are made, you will probably lose the medical insurance that came with your job if you discontinue your employment. In the US, If you are under age for medicare it may be extremely expensive or impossible to purchase new medical insurance.

Can I get social security disability?

Social security disability is for individuals who are permanently and completely disabled, and unable to engage in any gainful employment. Because the criteria are so strict, the process often takes a long time and many patients with Parkinson's disease are denied disability benefits the first time they apply. The key is to be persistent and reapply if you meet eligibility criteria. An attorney who specializes in social security disability can help.

I developed Parkinson's disease five years ago. I'm worried about the emotional impact the disease might have on my spouse.

Studies have demonstrated that the amount and type of stress experienced by a caregiver progresses and changes with each stage of the disease[19]. Caregiver stress is relatively low when the patient is in the first two stages of disease, although worry begins to emerge in stage II. When the patient is in stage III, caregivers experience increased tension and frustration, often stemming from communication problems and role conflict.

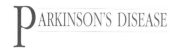
PARKINSON'S DISEASE

In stages IV and V, caregivers experience increased stress due to economic burdens, lack of resources, and feelings of manipulation. These stressors are very real and can have a profound impact on the patient, the caregiver, and their relationship.

Support groups, respite care, educational resources, and professional services may help to reduce strain on family members of PD patients. A social worker or psychologist may be of benefit to provide support and counseling. If possible, it is usually helpful for the caregiver to maintain independent activities and friends. Scheduled breaks from caregiving are also valuable. Expectations placed on the caregiver must be realistic and not overwhelming. Although many caregivers attempt to put forth superhuman efforts, this may cause more problems than it solves. It is often better to provide additional help as offered in an assisted care living facility or nursing home.

Should I take vitamins?

No vitamin is known to provide benefit for Parkinson's disease. Although there is interest as to whether vitamin E might slow the progression of PD, studies to date have not provided evidence that it does so [20]. We usually suggest that PD patients take a single multivitamin each day as we recommend for everyone.

What foods should I eat now that I've been diagnosed with Parkinson's disease?

Dietary protein interferes with the absorption of levodopa from the gut and its transport into the brain [21]. However, only patients with advanced disease who are very sensitive to small changes in levodopa absorption need to be concerned about this. Most patients should simply concentrate on eating a healthy diet. Increased fiber, fruits, and vegetables help prevent constipation. There is a tendency for patients to lose weight over time, so individuals of normal weight should strive to maintain it. Obese individuals will want to prudently lose weight so that mobility can be maintained as the disease progresses. Overly aggressive or quick weight loss should be avoided. Special low protein, protein redistributed, or balanced protein diets may help patients with advanced disease who find that they lose medication benefit when they eat a meal that includes protein. It is still important to take in enough protein to maintain overall health. We recommend consultation with a dietitian for patients who might benefit from a protein-modified diet.

How are new medications developed?

Research is what creates new and better treatments. Research that involves chemicals and cells in laboratories is called basic research and research that involves people is called clinical research. Promising new medications are initially discovered and developed in research laboratories. The medication is then tested in animals. If the medication is demonstrated to be safe and effective in animals, it may be tested in people.

In the initial phase of clinical research, the medication is evaluated in normal individuals who volunteer to be part of the testing program. If the medication is demonstrated to be safe in normal volunteers, it may then be tested in patients.

In sophisticated clinical trials, patients consent to receive pills that could be the real medication being tested or a fake (placebo) that contains no active medication. The reason this is done is because patients improve when they receive a placebo. This is called the placebo effect. In part, the placebo effect is due to psychological factors and in part due to the way patients are evaluated. Because of this, if only the real medication were given, doctors could not tell if improvement was really an effect of the medication or due to the placebo effect. We therefore compare the improvement in patients who received the real medication to the improvement in patients who received placebo. If the real medication provided more improvement than the placebo, we know it is the difference in improvement that is due to the medication because everything else was handled in exactly the same way. If both groups improve the same amount then the medication did not provide any benefit.

I do not want to take a placebo.

Clinical studies that include a placebo are designed to minimize patient discomfort and risk. Some studies are for patients with very early disease, before treatment is required. In these studies, patients have the luxury of being able to take a placebo because there is minimal disability and other medications are not needed. Other studies are designed for patients who are on antiparkinsonian medications and need them to maintain benefit.

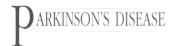
In these clinical trials the placebo (or medication under study) is added to the medications the patient is already taking.

Most clinical trials are designed for patients who are doing reasonably well or for those patients who are not doing well but for whom additional benefit cannot be achieved with currently available treatments. Although many patients improve in clinical trials you cannot count on getting better. If you are in need of more medication and would be unhappy if you stayed the same through the trial, you should not enter the study until your medications have been adjusted and you are doing better. Of course, there are many different study designs, and if your other antiparkinsonian medications can be increased during the trial, there may be even less concern regarding a placebo. Discuss the details of the study with your doctor.

Should I participate in a clinical trial?

This is a very individual decision. However, the value of clinical trials cannot be underestimated. Clinical trials allow new medications and procedures to be tested and hopefully approved for patient use. We are able to use the medications we have now because other patients participated in the clinical trials needed to assess these medications. You may participate in a trial of a medication that will help you and others later on. This is one way to play an active role in fighting the disease. We also find that we get to know our patients who participate in clinical trials very well because we see them frequently. There is usually no charge for the care you receive in a clinical trial.

Are there reasons not to participate in clinical trials?

Some clinical trials are easier than others. They differ in their duration, frequency of visits, and how long each evaluation takes. Some may be too demanding for you.

In addition, all medications have potential side-effects and it is possible to experience a side effect in a clinical trial. There is usually a mechanism built into the study to deal with this possibility. The medication might be discontinued or the dose lowered. In some cases the side effect is treated with another medication. The further along a drug is in its clinical testing the more that is known about it. Conversely, there may be less known about a medication when it is first tested in patients. Ask your doctor to put these issues in perspective for you for the particular study you are considering.

I am interested in participating in a clinical trial. How do I do this?

Expert Movement Disorder Centers generally conduct the most clinical research. The information resource centers at the end of this chapter can refer you to an Expert Center and may also have information about national and local clinical trials. You may also want to call your local university medical school for the names and phone numbers of Movement Disorders experts in your area.

I am interested in donating money to research on Parkinson's disease.

Movement Disorder Centers and national organizations are delighted to accept donations to support research.

What else?

It is very important to keep a positive mental outlook. Do your part to eat right, exercise, and get enough sleep. Find a good doctor who knows a lot about Parkinson's disease and whom you like and trust. Do what you can to support research.

Tremendous advances have been made in the recent past and the future looks extremely bright. An understanding of what causes the disease is close at hand. Understanding the cause will lead to a cure.

REFERENCES

Chapter 1 references

1.   Parkinson J. An essay on the shaking palsy. London; Sherwood, Neely & Jones 1817, 66.

2.   Wendell CM, Hauser RA, Nagaria MH, Sanchez-Ramos J, Zesiewicz TA. Chief complaints of patients with Parkinson's disease. Neurology 1999;52(Suppl 2):A90.

3.   Duvoisin RC. History of parkinsonism. Pharmacology and Therapeutics 1987;32:1-17.

4.   Martilla RJ, Rinne UK. Epidemiological approaches to the etiology of Parkinson's disease. Acta Neurol Scand 1989;126:13-18.

5.   Martilla RJ, Rinne UK. Epidemiology of Parkinson's disease in Finland. Acta Neurol Scand 1976;53(2);81-102.

6.   Lilienfeld DE, Chan E, Ehland J, Godbold J, Landrigan PH, Marsh G, Perl DP. Two decades of increasing mortality from Parkinson's disease among the US elderly. Arch Neurol 1990;47:731-734.

7.   Tanner CM, Ben-Shlomo Y. Epidemiology of Parkinson's disease. Adv Neurol 1999;80:153-159.

8.   Rajput AH, Offord K, Beard CM, Kurland LT. Epidemiology of Parkinsonism: incidence, classification, and mortality. Ann Neurol 1984;16:278-282.

9.   Ben-Shlomo Y, Sieradzan K. Idiopahtic Parkinosn's disease: epidemiology, diagnosis, and management. Br. J Gen Pract 1995;45:261-268.

10. Bharucha NE, Bharucha EP, Bharucha AE, Bhise AV, Schoenberg BS. Prevalence of Parkinson's disease in the Parsi community of Bombay, India. Arch Neurol 1988;45:1321-1323.

11. Melcon MO, Anderson DW, Vergara RH, Rocca WA. Prevalence of Parkinson's Disease in Junin, Buenos Aires Province, Argentina. Mov Disord 1997;12:197-205.

12. Morgante L, Rocca WA, DiRosa AE et al. Prevalence of Parkinson's disease and other types of parkinsonism: a door-to-door survey in three Sicilian municipalities. Neurology 1992;42:1901-1907.

13. Kessler II. Epidemiologic studies of Parkinson's disease. American J of Epi 1972;95:308-318.

14. Cosnett JE, Bill PL. Parkinson's disease in blacks. Observations on epidemiology in Natal. South African Medical Journal 1988;73:281-3.

15. Schoenberg BS, Anderson DW, Haerer AF. Prevalence of Parkinson's disease in the biracial population of Copiah County, Mississippi. Neurology 1985;35:841-845.

16. Mayeux R, Marder K, Cote L, Denaro J, Hemenegildo N, Mejia H, Tang MX, Lantigua R, Wilder D, Gurland B, Hauser A. The frequency of idiopathic Parkinson's disease by age, ethnic group, and sex in northern Manhattan, 1988-1993. Am J Epidemiol 1995;142:820-827.

17. Manyam BV. Paralysis agitans and levodopa in "Ayurveda": ancient Indian medical treatise. Movement Disorders 1990;5:47-8.

18. Ballard PA, Tetrud JW, Langston JW. Permanent human parkinsonism due to 1-methyl-4-phenyl-1,2,3,6-tetrahydropyridine (MPTP): seven cases. Neurology 1985;35:949-956.

19. Hoehn MM. The natural history of Parkinson's disease in the pre-levodopa and post-levodopa eras. In: Cedarbaum JM, Gancher ST eds. Neurologic Clinics. Philadelphia PA: W.B. Saunders and Company 1992;331.

20. Tanner CM, Thelen JA, Offord KP, Rademacher D, Goetz CG, Kurland LT. Relationship of age at diagnosis to survival in Parkinson's disease (PD). Mov Disord 1992;7:104.

21. Wichman T, DeLong M. Pathophysiology of parkinsonian motor abnormalities. In: Narabayashi H, Nagatsu T, Yanagisawa N, Mizuno Y. Advances in Neurology New York: Raven Press 1993;53-60.

22. Gibb WRG. Neuropathology of movement disorders. J Neurol Neurosurg Psych 1989;55-67.

23. Hirsch E, Graybiel AM, Agid YA. Melanized dopaminergic neurons are differentially susceptible to degeneration in Parkinson's disease. Nature 1988;334:345-348.

24. Fearnley JM, Lees AJ. Ageing and Parkinson's disease: substantia nigra regional selectivity. Brain 1991;114:2283-2301.

25. Poewe WH, Wenning GK. The natural history of Parkinson's disease. Ann Neurol 1998;44(Suppl 1):S1-S9.

26. Spillantini MG, Schmidt ML, Lee VM et al. Alpha-synuclein in Lewy bodies. Nature 1997;388:839-840.

27. Richards M, Marder K, Cote L, Mayeux R. Reliability of symptom onset assessment in Parkinson's disease. Mov Disord 1994;9:340-342.

28. Aarsland D, Larsen JP, Lim NG, Janvin C, Karlsen D, Tandberg E, Cummings JL. Range of neuropsychiatric disturbances in patients with Parkinson's disease. J Neurol Neurosurg Psychiatry 1999;67:492-496.

29. Nagatsu T. Biochemical aspects of Parkinson's disease. In: Narabayashi H, Nagatsu T, Yanagisawa N, Mizuno Y. Advances in Neurology New York: Raven Press 1993;165-174.

30. Agid Y, Cervera P, Hirsch E, Javoy-Agid F, Lehericy S, Raisman R, Ruberg M. Biochemistry of Parkinson's disease 28 years later: a critical review. Movement Disorders 1989;4:S126-44.

31. Goldstein M, Lieberman A. The role of the regulatory enzymes of catecholamine synthesis in Parkinson's disease. Neurology 1992;42:8-12

32. Sibley DR, Monsma FJ Jr. Molecular biology of dopamine receptors. Trends Pharmacol Sci 1992;13:61-9.

33. Kebabian JW, Calne DB. Multiple receptors for dopamine. Nature 1979;277:93-96.

34. Calne DB. Treatment of Parkinson's disease. New Eng J Med 1993;3239:1021-1027.

35. Brooks DJ, Ibanez V, Sawle GV, et al. Differing patterns of striatal 18F-dopa uptake in Parkinson's disease, multiple system atrophy, and progressive supranuclear palsy. Ann Neurol 1990;28:547-55.

36. Brucke T, Kornhuber J, Angelberger P, Asenbaum S, Frassine H, Podreka I. SPECT imaging of dopamine and serotonin transporters with [123I] beta-CIT. Binding kinetics in the human brain. J Neurol Transm 1993;94:137-46.

Chapter 2 references

1. Marder K, Tang MX, Meijia H, et al. Risk of Parkinson's disease among first-degree relatives: a community-based study. Neurology 1996;47:155-160.

2. Ward CD, Duvoisin RC, Ince SE, et al. Parkinson's disease in 65 pairs of twins and in a set of quadruplets. Neurology 1983:33:815-824.

3. Johnson WH, Hodge WE, Duvoisin R. Twin studies and the genetics of Parkinson's disease-a reappraisal. Mov Disord 1990;5:187-194.

4. Tanner CM, Ottman R, Ellenberg JH, et al. Parkinson's disease in twins: an etiologic study. JAMA 1999;281:341-346.

5. Piccini P, Burn DJ, Ceravolo R, et al. The role of inheritance in sporadic Parkinson's disease: evidence from a longitudinal study of dopaminergic function in twins. Ann Neurol 1999;45:577-582.

6. Sveinbjornsd`ttir S, Hicks AA, Jonsson T, et al. Familial aggregation of Parkinson's disease in Iceland. N Engl J Med. 2000;343:1765-1770.

7. Golbe LI, Di Iorio G, Sanges G, et al. Clinical genetic analysis of Parkinson's disease in the Contursi kindred. Ann Neurol 1996;40:767-775.

8. Polymeropoulos MH, Higgins JJ, Golbe LI, et al. Mapping of a gene for Parkinson's disease in the Contursi kindred. Science 1996;274:1265-1269.

9. Polymeropoulos MH, Lavedan C, Leroy E. Mutation in the a-Synuclein gene identified in families with Parkinson's disease. Science 1997;276:2045-2047.

10. Markopoulou K, Wszolek ZK, Pfeiffer RF. A Greek-American kindred with autosomal dominant, levodopa-responsive parkinsonism and anticipation. Ann Neurol 1995;38:373-378.

11. Krhger R, Kuhn W, Muller T, et al. Ala30Pro mutation in the gene encoding alpha-synuclein in Parkinson's disease. Nat Genet 1998;18:106-108.

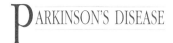

12. Lashuel HA, Petre BM, Wall J, Simon M, Nowak RJ, Walz T, Lansbury PT Jr. Alpha-synuclein, especially the Parkinson's disease-associated mutants, forms pore-like annular and tubular protofibrils. J Mol Biol 2002;322:1089-1092.

13. Spillantini MG, Schmidt ML, Lee VM, et al. Alpha-synuclein in Lewy bodies. Nature 1997;388:839-840.

14. Lotharius J, Brundin P. Impaired dopamine storage resulting from alpha-synuclein mutations may contribute to the pathogenesis of Parkinson's disease. Hum Mol Genet 2002;11:2395-2407.

15. Conway KA, Rochet JC, Bieganski RM, Lansbury PT Jr. Kinetic stabilization of the alpha-synuclein protofibril by a dopamine-alpha-synuclein adduct. Science 2001;294:1346-1349.

16. Betarbet R, Sherer TB, MacKenzie G, Garcia-Osuna M, Panov AV, Greenamyre JT. Chronic systemic pesticide exposure reproduces features of Parkinson's disease. Nat Neurosci 2000;3:1301-1306.

17. Uversky VN, Li J, Bower K, Fink AL. Synergistic effects of pesticides and metals on the fibrillation of alpha-synuclein: implications for Parkinson's disease. Neurotoxicology 2002;23:527-536.

18. Feany MB, Bender WW. A Drosophila model of Parkinson's disease. Nature 2000;404:394-398.

19. Masliah E, Rockenstein E, Veinbergs I, et al. Dopaminergic loss and inclusion body formation in alpha-synuclein mice: implications for neurodegenerative disorders. Science 2000;287:1265-1269.

20. Auluck PK, Chan HY, Trojanowski JQ, Lee VM, Bonini NM. Chaperone suppression of alpha-synuclein toxicity in a Drosophila model for Parkinson's disease. Science 2002;295:865-868.

21. Auluck PK, Bonini NM. Pharmacological prevention of Parkinson disease in Drosophila. Nat Med 2002;8:1185-1186.

22. Ishikawa A, Tsuji S. Clinical analysis of 17 patients in 12 Japanese families with autosomal recessive type juvenile parkinsonism. Neurology 1996;47:160-166.

23. Yamamura Y, Sobue I, Ando K et al. Paralysis agitans of early onset with marked diurnal fluctuation of symptoms. Neurology 1983;23;239-244.

24. Takahashi H, Ohama E, Suzuki S et al. Familial juvenile parkinsonism: clinical and pathologic study in a family. Neurology 1994;44:437-441.

25. Lhcking CB, Durr A, Bonifati V, et al. Association between early onset Parkinson's disease and mutations in the parkin gene. French Parkinson's Disease Genetics Study Group. N Engl J Med. 2000;342:1560-1567.

26. Kitada T, Asakawa H, Hattori N et al. Mutations in the parkin gene cause autosomal recessive juvenile parkinsonism. Nature 1998;392:605-608.

27. West A, Periquet M, Lincoln S, et al. Complex relationship between Parkin mutations and Parkinson disease. Am J Med Genet 2002;114:584-591.

28. Tanaka K, Suzuki T, Chiba T, Shimura H, Hattori N, Mizuno Y. J Mol Med 2001;79:482-494.

29. Bennett MC, Bishop JF, Leng, Chock PB, Chase TN, Mouradian MM. Degradation of alpha-synuclein by proteasome. J Biol Chem 1999;274:33855-33858.

30. Leroy E, Boyer R, Auburger G, et al. The ubiquitin pathway in Parkinson's disease. Nature 1998;395:451-452.

31. West AB, Zimprich A, Lockhart PJ, et al. Refinement of the PARK3 locus on chromosome 2p13 and the analysis of 14 candidate genes. Eur J Hum Genet 2001;9:659-666.

32. DeStefano AL, Lew MF, Golbe LI, et al. PARK3 influences age at onset in Parkinson disease: a genome scan in the GenePD study. Am J Hum Genet 2002;70:1085-1089.

33. Earle KM. Studies on Parkinson's disease including x-ray fluorescence spectroscopy of formalin fixed brain tissue. J Neuropath Exp Neurol 1968;27:1-14.

34. Kim KS, Choi SY, Kwon HY, Won MH, Kang TC, Kang JH. Aggregation of alpha-synuclein induced by the Cu,Zn-superoxide dismutase and hydrogen peroxide system. Free Radic Biol Med 2002;32:544-550.

35. Hashimoto M, Hsu LJ, Xia Y, Takeda A, Sisk A, Sundsmo M, Masliah E. Oxidative stress induces amyloid-like aggregate formation of NACP/alpha-synuclein in vitro. Neuroreport 1999;10:717-721.

36. Sian J, Dexter DT, Lees AJ, et al. Alterations in glutathione levels in Parkinson's disease and other neurodegenerative disorders affecting basal ganglia. Ann Neurol 1994;36:348-355.

37. Gerlach M, Ben-Shachar D, Riederer P, Youdim MBH. Altered brain metabolism of iron as a cause of neurodegenerative diseases? J Neurochem 1994;63:793-807.

38. Youdim MB, Ben-Shachar D, Riederer P. The enigma of neuromelanin in Parkinson's disease substantia nigra. J Neurol Trans 1994;43:113-22.

39. Kalra J, Rajput AH, Mantha SV, Chaudhary AK, Prasad K. Oxygen free radical producing activity of polymorphonuclear leukocytes in patients with Parkinson's disease. Molecular and Cellular Biochemistry 1992;112:181-6.

40. Przedborski S, Kostic V, Jackson-Lewis V, et al. Transgenic mice with increased Cu/Zn-superoxide dismutase activity are resistant to N-methyl-4-phenyl-1,2,3,6-tetrahydropyridine-induced neurotoxicity. J Neurosci 1992;12:1658-1667.

41. Hirsch EC. Why are nigral catecholaminergic neurons more vulnerable than other cells in Parkinson's disease? Ann Neurol 1992;32:S88-93.

42. Zhang P, Damier P, Hirsch EC, et al. Preferential expression of superoxide dismutase messenger RNA in melanized neurons in human mesencephalon. Neurosci 1993;55:167-175.

43. Checkoway H, Costa LG, Woods JS, Castoldi AF, Lund BO, Swanson PD. Peripheral blood cell activities of monoamine oxidase B and superoxide dismutase in Parkinson's disease. J Neural Trans 1992;4:283-90.

44. Davis GC, Williams AC, Markey SP, Ebert MH, Caine ED, Reichert CM, Kopin IJ. Chronic parkinsonism secondary to intravenous injection of meperidine analogues. Psychiatry Research 1979;1:249-254.

45. Ballard PA, Tetrud JW, Langston JW. Permanent human parkinsonism due to 1-methyl-4-phenyl-1,2,3,6 tetrahydropyridine (MPTP): seven cases. Neurology 1985;35:949-956.

46. Semchuk KM, Love EJ, Lee RG. Parkinson's disease: a test of the multifactorial etiologic hypothesis. Neurology 1993;43:1173-1180.

47. Davey GP, Tipton KF, Murphy MP. Uptake and accumulation of 1-methyl-4-phenylpyridinium by rat liver mitochondria measured using an ion-selective electrode. Biochem Med J 1992;288:439-43.

48. Schapira AH, Mann VM, Cooper JM, et al. Anatomic and disease specificity of NADH CoQ1 reductase (complex 1) deficiency in Parkinson's disease. J Neurochem 1990;55:2142-2145.

49. Haas RH, Nsairian F, Nakano K, Ward D, Pay M, Hill R, Shults CW. Low platelet mitochondrial complex I and complex II/III activity in early untreated Parkinson's disease. Ann Neurol 1995;37:714-22.

50. Kessler II. Epidemiologic studies of Parkinson's disease. 3. A community-based survey. American Journal of Epidemiology 1972;96:242-54.

51. Hernan MA, Takkouche B, Caamano-Isorna F, Gestal-Otero JJ. A meta-analysis of coffee drinking, cigarette smoking, and the risk of Parkinson's disease. Ann Neurol 2002;52:276-84

52. Carlsson A, Winblad B. Influence of age and time interval between death and autopsy on dopamine and 3-methoxytyramine levels in human basal ganglia. J Neural Transm 1976; 38:271-276.

53. Purjol J, Junque C, Vendrell P, Grau JM, Capdevila A. Reduction of the substantia nigra width and motor decline in aging and Parkinson's disease. Arch Neurol 1992;49:1119-1122.

54. Calne DB, Peppard RF. Aging of the nigrostriatal pathway in humans. Can J Neurol Sci 1987;14:424-427.

55. Fearnley JM, Lees AJ. Aging and Parkinson's disease: substantia nigra regional selectivity. Brain 1991;114:2283-301.

56. Neuman RP, LeWitt PA, Jaffe M, Calne DB, Larsen TA. Motor function in the normal aging population; treatment with levodopa. Neurology 1985;35:571-573.

57. Schwartz J, Elizan T. Search for viral particles and virus-specific products in idiopathic Parkinson's disease brain material. Ann Neurol 1979;6:261-263.

58. Martilla RJ, Rinne UK, Halonen P, Madden DL, Sever JL. Herpes viruses and parkinsonism. Arch Neurol 1981;38:19-21. Nat Med 2002;8:1185-1186.

Chapter 3 references

1. Schou M, Baastrup PC, Grof P, Weis P, Angst J. Pharmacological and clinical problems of lithium prophylaxis. Br J Psych 1970;116:615-619.

2. Yamadori A, Albert M. Involuntary movement disorder caused by methyldopa. N Eng J Med 1972;286:610.

3. Rajput AH, Rozdilsky B, Hornykiewicz O et al. Reversible drug-induced parkinsonism. Arch Neurol 1982;39:644-646.

4. Logan WJ, Freeman JM. Pseudodegenerative disease due to diphenylhydantoin intoxication. Arch Neurol 1969;21:631-637.

5. Karas BJ, Wilder BJ, Hammond EJ et al. Treatment of valproate tremors. Neurology 1983;33:1380-1382.

6. Gibb WRG. Accuracy in the clinical diagnosis of parkinsonian syndromes. Postgraduate Med Jour 1988;64:345-351.

7. Ballard PA, Tetrud JW, Langston JW. Permanent human parkinsonism due to 1-methyl-4-phenyl-1,2,3,6-tetrahydropyridine (MPTP): seven cases. Neurology 1985;35:949-956.

8. Tolosa ES, Santamaria J. Parkinsonism and basal ganglia infarcts. Neurology 1984;34:1516-8.

9. Ferbert A, Gerwig M. Tremor due to stroke. Movement Disorders 1993;8:179-182.

10. Duvoisin RC, Yahr MD. Encephalitis and parkinsonism. Arch Neurol 1965;12:227-239.

11. Ziegler LH. Follow-up studies on persons who have had epidemic encephalitis. JAMA 1928;91:138-141.

12. Martland JS. Punch drunk. JAMA 1928;91:1103-7.

13. Corselis JAN, Bruton CJ, Freeman-Browne D. The aftermath of boxing. Psychol Med 1973;3:270-303.

14. Larsen TA, Calne DB. Essential tremor. Clin Neuropharmacol 1983;6:185-206.

15. Critchley M. Observations on essential (heredofamilial) tremor. Brain 1949;72:113-39.

16. Larson T, Sjogren T. Essential tremor. A clinical and genetic population study. Acta Psychiatr Neurol Scand 1960;36:1-176.

17. Koller WC, Busenbark K, Gray C, Hassanein RS, Dubinsky R. Classification of essential tremor. Clin Neurophar 1992;15:81-87.

18. Wilson SAK. Progressive lenticular degeneration: a familial nervous disease associated with cirrhosis of the liver. Brain 1912;34:295-507.

19. Levine IM, Estes JW, Looney JM. Hereditary neurological disease with acanthocytosis. A new syndrome. Arch Neurol 1968;19:403-409.

20. Aminoff MJ. Acanthocytosis and neurological disease. Brain 1972;95:749-760.

21. Sotaniemi KA. Chorea acanthocythosis-neurologic disease with acanthocytosis. Acta Neurol Scand 1983;68:53-56.

22. Huntington G. On Chorea. Lea and Blanchard, Philadelphia, Medical and Surgical Reporter 1872;26:317.

23. Hayden MR. Huntington's chorea. New York, Springer-Verlag, 1981.

24. Huntington's Disease Collaborative Research Group. A novel gene containing a trinucleotide repeat that is expanded and unstable on Huntington's disease chromosomes. Cell 1993;72:971-983.

25. Klawans HL, Weiner WJ. The pharmacology of choreatic movement disorder. Prog Neurobiol 1976;6:49-80.

26. Steele JC, Richardson JC, Olszewski J. Progressive supranuclear palsy. Arch Neurol 1964;10:333-359.

27. Golbe LI, Davis PH, Schoenberg BS, Duvoisin RC. Prevalence and natural history of progressive supranuclear palsy. Neurology 1988;38:1031-1034.

28. Jankovic J, Friedman DI, Pirozzolo FJ, McCrary JA. Progressive supranuclear palsy: motor, neurobehavioral, and neuro-ophthalmic findings. In: Streifler MB, Korczyn AD, Melamed E, Youdim MBH, Advances in Neurology; Raven Press, New York, 1990.

29. Fukushima-Kudo J, Fukushima K, Tashiro K. Rigidity and dorsiflexion of the neck in progressive supranuclear palsy and the interstitial nucleus of Cajal. J Neurol Neurosurg Psychiatry 1987;50:1197-1203.

30. Pillon B, Dubois B, Lhermitte F, Agid Y. Heterogeneity of cognitive impairment in progressive supranuclear palsy, Parkinson's disease, and Alzheimer's disease. Neurology 1986;36:1179-1185.

31. Oppenheimer DR. Diseases of the basal ganglia, cerebellum and motorneurons. In Blackwood W, Corsellis JAN Eds: Greenfield's Neuropathology. London, Edward Arnold 1976:608-651.

32. Quinn N. Multiple system atrophy-the nature of the beast. J Neurol Neurosurg Psychiatry 1989;52:78-79.

33. Shy GM, Drager GA. A neurological syndrome associated with orthostatic hypotension: a clinical-pathological study. Arch Neurol 1960;2:511-527.

34. Rajput AH, Rozdilsky B. Dysautonomia in parkinsonism: a clinicopathological study. J Neurol Neurosurg Psychiatry 1976;39:1092-1100.

35. Lees AJ, Bannister R. The use of lisuride in the treatment of multiple system atrophy with autonomic failure (Shy-Drager syndrome). J Neurol Neurosurg Psychiatry 1981;44:347-351.

36. Dejerine J, Thomas A. L'atrophie olivo-ponto-cerebelleuses. Nouv Iconogr Salpet 1900;13:330-370.

37. Berciano J. Olivopontocerebellar atrophy. J Neurol Sci 1982;53:253-272.

38. Koeppen AH, Barron KD. The neuropathology of olivopontocerebellar atrophy. In: Duvoisin RC, Plaitakis A Eds: The Olivopontocerebellar Atrophies. New York, Raven Press 1984:13-38.

39. Huang YP, Plaitakis A. Morphological changes of olivopontocerebellar atrophy in computed tomography and comments on its pathogenesis. In Duvoisin RC, Plaitakis A Eds: The Olivopontocerebellar Atrophies. New York, Raven Press 1984:39-85.

40. Adams RD, Van Bogaert L, Van Der Eecken H. Striatonigral degeneration. J Neuropath Exp Neruol 1964;23:584-608.

41. Takei Y, Samuels NS. Striatonigral degeneration: a form of multiple system atrophy with clinical parkinsonism. In: Zimmerman HM Ed: Progress in Neuropathology Vol 2. New York, Grune and Stratton 1973, 217-251.

42. Reibeiz JJ, Kolodny EH, Richardson E. Corticodentatonigral degeneration with neuronal achromasia. Arch Neurol 1968;18:20-33.

43. Riley DE, Lang AE, Lewis A, et al. Cortical-basal ganglionic degeneration. Neurology 1990;40:1203-1212.

44. Case records of the Massachusetts General Hospital. N Engl J Med 1985;313:739-748.

45. Louis ED, Goldman JE, Powers JM, Fahn S. Parkinsonian features of eight pathologically diagnosed cases of diffuse Lewy body disease. Movement Disorders 1994;10:188-94.

46. Hansen LA, Galasko D. Lewy body disease. Current Opinion in Neurology & Neurosurgery. 1992;5:889-94.

Chapter 4 references

1. Calne DB, Stoessl AJ. Early parkinsonism. Clinical Neuropharmacology 1986;9:S3-8.

2. Calne DB, Snow BJ, Lee C. Criteria for diagnosing Parkinson's disease. Ann Neurol 1992;32:S125-127.

3. Martilla RJ, Rinne UK. Epidemiology of Parkinson's disease in Finland. Acta Neurol Scand 1976;53:81-102.

4. Gudmundsson KRA. A clinical survey of parkinsonism in Iceland. Acta Neurol Scand 1967;43(suppl):9-61.

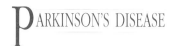

5. Nobrega FT, Glattre E, Kurland LT, Okazaki H. Comments on the epidemiolgy of parkinsonism including prevalence and incidence statistics for Rochester, Minnesota, 1935-1966. In: Barbeau A, Brunette JR, eds. Progress in Neurogenetics. Proceedings of the Second International Congress of Neurogenetics and Neuro-Ophthalmology. Amsterdam: Excerpta Medica, 1969.

6. Gibb WRG, Lees AJ. The clinical phenomenon of akathisia. J Neur Neurosurg Psych 1986;49:861-866.

7. Hoehn MM, Yahr MD. Parkinsonism: onset, progression and mortality. Neurology 1967;17:427-442.

8. Mutch WJ, Dingwall-Fordyce I, Downie AW, Paterson JG, Roy SK. Parkinson's disease in a Scottish city. Br Med J 1986;292:534-536.

9. Schrag A, Ben-Shlono Y, Brown R, Marsden CD, Quinn N. Young-onset Parkinson's disease revisited - clinical features, natural history, and mortality. Mov Disord 1998;13:885-894.

10. Rosati G, Granieri E, Pinna L, et al. The risk of Parkinson's disease in Mediterranean people. Neurology 1980;30:250-255.

11. Harada H, Nishikawa S, Takahaski K. Epidemiology of Parkinson's disease in a Japanese city. Arch Neurol 1983;40:151-154.

12. Gibb WRG, Lees AJ. A comparison of clinical and pathological features of young- and old-onset Parkinson's disease. Neurology 1988;38:1402-1406.

13. Aarsland D, Larsen JP, Lim NG, et al. Range of neuropsychiatric disturbnaces in patients with Parkinson's disease. J Neurol Neurosurg Psychiatry 1999;67:492-496.

14. Juncos JL. Management of psychotic aspects of Parkinson's disease. J Clin Psychiatry 1999;60(suppl 8): 42-53.

15. Cummings JL. Behavioral complications of drug treatment of Parkinson's disease. J Am Geriatr Soc 1991;39:708-716.

16. Factor SA, Molho ES, Podskalny GD, et al. Parkinson's disease: drug-induced psychiatric states. Adv Neurol 1995;65:115-138.

17. Peyser CE, maimark D, Zuniga R, et al. Psychoses in Parkinson's disease. Semin Clin Neuropsychiatry 1998;3:41-50.

18. Diagnostic and Statistical Manual of Mental Disorders, fourth edition. American Psychiatric Association Washington D.C. 1994;134.

19. Brown RG, Marsden CD. How common is dementia in Parkinson's disease? The Lancet 1984;56;1262-1265.

20. Lieberman A, Dziatolowski M, Kupersmith M, Serby M, Goodgold A, Korein J, and Goldstein M. Dementia in Parkinson's disease. Ann Neurol 1979;6:355-359.

21. Hurtig HI, Trojanowski JQ, Galvin J, et al. Alpha-synuclein cortical Lewy bodies correlate with dementia in Parkinson's disease. Neurology 2000;54:1916-1921.

22. Agid Y, Ruberg M, Dubois B et al. Parkinson's disease and dementia. Clin Neuropharm 1986;9:S22-36.

23. Cummings JL. Depression and Parkinson's disease: a review. Am J Psychiatry 1992;149:443-454.

24. Mayeux R, Stern Y, Williams JBW, Cote L, Frantz A, Dyrenfurth I. Clinical and biochemical features of depression in Parkinson's disease. Am J Psychiatry 1986;143:756-759.

25. Awerbuch GI. Autonomic functions in the early stages of Parkinson's disease. Intern J Neuroscience 1992;64:7-14.

26. Turkka JT, Tolonen U, Myllyla VV. Cardiovascular reflexes in Parkinson's disease. European Neurology 1987;26:104-12.

27. Langston JW, Forno LS. The hypothalamus in Parkinson's disease. Ann Neurol 1978;3:129-133.

28. Ondo WG, Dat Vuong K, Khan H, Atassi F, Kwak C, Jankovic J. Daytime sleepiness and other sleep disorders in Parkinson's disease. Neurology 2001;57:1392-1396.

29. Frucht S, Rogers JD, Greene PE, Gordon MF, Fahn S. Falling asleep at the wheel: motor vehicle mishaps in persons taking pramipexole and ropinirole. Neurology 1999;52:1908-1910.

30. Parkinson Study Group. Pramipexole vs levodopa as initial treatment for Parkinson disease: a randomized controlled trial. JAMA 2000;284:1931-1938.

31. Rascol O, Brooks DJ, Korczyn AD, De Deyn PP, Clarke CE, Lang AE. A five-year study of the incidence of dyskinesia in patients with early Parkinson's disease who were treated with ropinirole or levodopa. N Engl J Med 2000;342:1484-1491.

32. Rye DB, Bliwise DL, Dihenia B, Gurecki P. Daytime sleepiness in Parkinson's disease. J Sleep Res 2000;9:63-69.

33. Comella C, Nardine T, Diederich N, Stebbins G. Sleep-related violence, injury, and REM sleep behavior disorder in Parkinson's disease. Neurology 1998;51:526-529.

34. Schenck CH, Bundlie SR, Mahowald MW. Delayed emergence of a parkinsonian disorder in 38% of 29 older men diagnosed with idiopathic rapid eye movement sleep behavior disorder. Neurology 1996;46:388-393.

35. Arnulf I, Konofal E, Merino-Andreu M, et al. Parkinson's disease and sleepiness: An integral part of PD. Neurology 2002;58:1019-1024.

36. Laihinen A, Alihanka J, Raitasuo S, Rinne UK. Sleep movements and associated autonomic nervous activities in patients with Parkinson's disease. Acta Neurol Scand 1987;76:64-68.

37. Mouret J. Differences in sleep in patients with Parkinson's disease. Electroencephalography & Clinical Neurophysiology. 1975;38:653-7.

38. Hoehn M. Commentary: Parkinsonism: onset, progression, and mortality. Neurology 1998;50(8):38.

39. Poewe WH, Wenning GK. The natural history of Parkinson's disease. Ann Neurol 1998;44(Suppl 1):S1-S9.

40. Fahn S, Elton RL, Members of the UPDRS Development Committee. Unified Parkinson's disease rating scale. In: Fahn S, Marsden CD, Calne DB, Goldstein M, Eds. Recent developments in Parkinson's disease. Vol 2. Florham Park, NJ: Macmillan Health Care Information 1987, 153-164.

Chapter 5 references

1. Fahn S. "On-off" phenomenon with levodopa therapy in parkinsonism. Clinical and pharmacologic correlates and the effect of intramuscular pyridoxine. Neurology 1974;24:431-441.

2. Marsden CD, Parkes JD. "On-off" effects in patients with Parkinson's disease on chronic levodopa therapy. Lancet 1976;1:292-296.

3. Sage JI, Mark M. The rationale for continuous dopaminergic stimulation in patients with Parkinson's disease (review). Neurology 1992;42:S23-8

4. Chase TN, Mouradian MM, Engber TM. Motor response complications and the function of striatal efferent systems. Neurology 1993;43:S23-27.

5. Muenter MD, Sharpless NS, Tyce GM, Darly FL. Patterns of dystonia ("I-D-I" and "D-I-D") in response to L-dopa therapy for Parkinson's disease. Mayo Clin Proc 1977;52:163-174.

6. Mones RJ, Elizan TS, Siegel GJ. Analysis of L-dopa induced dyskinesias in 51 patients with parkinsonism. J Neurol Neurosurg Psychiatry 1971;34:668-73.

7. McHale DM, Sage JI, Sonsalla PK, Vitagliano D. Complex dystonia of Parkinson's disease: clinical features and relation to plasma levodopa profile. Clinical Neuropharmacology 1990;13:164-170.

8. Poewe WH, Lees AJ, Stern GM. Low-dose L-dopa therapy in Parkinson's disease; a 6-year follow up. Neurology 1986;36:1528-1530.

9. Hauser RA, Zesiewicz TA, Factor SA, Guttman M, Weiner W. Clinical trials of add-on medications in Parkinson's disease: efficacy versus usefulness. Parkinsonism Rel Disord 1997;3:1-6.

10. Jenner P, Al-Barghouthy G, Smith L, et al. Initiation of entacapone with l-dopa further improves antiparkinsonian activity and avoids dyskinesia in the MPTP primate model of Parkinson's disease. Neurology 2002;58 (suppl 3):A374-A375.

11. Pearce RK, Banerji T, Jenner P, Marsden CD. De novo administration of ropinirole and bromocriptine induces less dyskinesia than levodopa in MPTP-treated marmosets. Mov Disord 1998;13:234-241.

12. Rascol O, Brooks DJ, Korczyn AD, et al. A five-year study of the incidence of dyskinesia in patients with early Parkinson's disease who were treated with ropinirole or levodopa. N Engl J Med 2000;342:1484-1491.

13. Parkinson Study Group. Pramipexole versus levodopa as initial treatment for Parkinson's disease: a randomized controlled trial. JAMA 2000;284:1931-1938.

14. Giladi N, McMahon D, Przedborski S, Flaster E, Guillory S, Kostic V, Fahn S. Motor blocks in Parkinson's disease. Neurology 1992;42:333-339.

Chapter 6 references

1.   Cotzias GC, Van Woert MH, Shiffer LM. Aromatic amino acids and modification of parkinsonism. N Engl J Med 1967;276:347-379.

2.   Carlsson A. The occurrence, distribution, and physiological role of catecholamines in the nervous system. Pharmacol Rev 1959;11:490-493.

3.   Ehringer, H, Hornykiewicz O. Vertelung von noradrenalin and dopamin (3-hydroxytyramin) im gehirn des menschen und ihr verhalten bei erkrankum gen des extrapyramidalen systems. Klin Wschr 1960;38:1236-1239.

4.   Cotzias GC, Papavasilou PS, Gellene R. Experimental treatment of parkinsonism with L-dopa. Neurology 1968;18:276-7.

5.   Bartholini GJ, Pletscher A. Effects of various decarboxylase inhibitors on the cerebral metabolism of dihydroxyphenylalanine. J Pharamacol 1969;21:323-324.

6.   Kurlan R, Rothfield AB, Woodward WR, Nutt JG, Miller C, Lichter D, and Shoulson I. Erratic gastric empting of levodopa may cause "random" fluctuations of parkinsonian mobility. Neurology 1988;48:419-421.

7.   Leon AS, Spiegel HE. The effect of antacid administration on the absorption and metabolism of levodopa. J Clinical Pharmacol 1972;12:263-267.

8.   Nutt JG, Fellman JH. Pharmacokinetics of levodopa. Clin Neuropharm 1984;7:35-49.

9.   Physicians Desk Reference 57th ed. Thompson PDR: Montvale, New Jersey, 2003.

10. Pahwa R, Lyons K, Marjama J, et al. Clinical experience with generic carbidopa/levodopa (G-L) in patients with Parkinson's disease. Neurology 1994;44(suppl 2):A244.

11. Pahwa R, Marjama J, McGuire D, et al. Pharmacokinetic comparison of Sinemet and Atamet (generic carbidopa/levodopa) a single dose study. Mov Disord 1996;11:427-430.

12. Pittner H, Stormann H, Enzenhofer R. Pharmacodynamic actions of midodrine, a new a-adrenergic stimulating agent, and its main metabolite, ST 1059. Arzneim Forsch 1976;26:2145-2154.

13. Goetz CG, Tanner CM, Klawans HL et al. Parkinson's disease and motor fluctuations: long-acting carbidopa/levodopa (CR4-Sinemet). Neurology 1987;37:875-878.

14. Yeh KC, August TF, Bush DF et al. Pharmacokinetics and bioavailability of Sinemet CR:a summary of human studies. Neurology 1989;39:S25-32.

15. Hutton JT, Morris JL. Long-acting carbidopa-levodopa in the management of moderate and advanced Parkinson's disease. Neurology 1992;42:51-56.

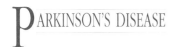
16. Rodnitzky R. The use of Sinemet CR in the management of mild to moderate Parkinson's disease. Neurology 1992;42 (suppl 1):44-50.

17. Jenner P, Al-Barghouthy G, Smith L, et al. Initiation of entacapone with l-dopa further improves antiparkinsonian activity and avoids dyskinesia in the MPTP primate model of Parkinson's disease. Neurology 2002;58 (suppl 3):A374-A375.

17b. Block G, Liss C, Reines S, Irr J, Nibbelink D, The CR First Study Group. Comparison of immediate-release and controlled release carbidopa/levodopa in Parkinson's disease. A multicenter 5-year study. Eur Neurol 1997;37:23-27.

18. Lees AJ. Madopar HBS (hydrodynamically balanced system) in the treatment of Parkinson's disease. In: Korczyn AD, Melamed E, Youdim MBH eds. Advances in Neurology New York: Raven Press, 1990:475-82.

19. Koller W. Pharmacologic treatment of parkinsonian tremor. Arch Neurol 1986;43:126-127.

20. Jenner P. The rationale for the use of dopamine agonists in Parkinson's disease. Neurology 1995;45:S6-12.

21. Montastruc, JL, Rascol O, Senard JM. Current status of dopamine agonists in Parkinson's disease management. Drugs 1993;46:384-393.

22. Langtry J, Clissold SP. Pergolide: a review of its pharmacological properties and therapeutic potential in Parkinson's disease. Drugs 1990;39:491-506.

23. Pritchett AM, Morrison JF, Edwards WD, Schaff HV, Connolly HM, Espinoza RE. Valvular heart disease in patients taking pergolide. Mayo Clinic Proc 2002;77:1280-1286.

24. Olanow CW, Fahn S, Muenter M. A multicenter double-blind placebo-controlled trial of pergolide as an adjunct to Sinemet in Parkinson's disease. Movement Disorders 1994;9:40-47.

25. Brefel C, Thalamus C, Rayet S, et al. Effect of food on the pharmacokinetics of ropinirole in parkinsonian patients. Br J Clin Pharmacol 1998:45:412-415.

26. Kreider M, Knox S, Gardiner D, Wheadon D. A multicenter double-blind study of ropinirole as an adjunct to L-dopa in Parkinson's disease. Neurology 1996;46 (Suppl):A475.

27. Wheadon DE, Wilson-Lynch K, Gardiner D, Kreider MS. Ropinirole, a non-ergoline D2 agonist, is effective in early parkinsonian patients not treated with L-dopa. Movement Disorders 1996;11(Suppl 1):162.

28. Rascol O on behalf of the Study Group. A double-blind L-dopa controlled study of ropinirole in de novo patients with Parkinson's disease. Mov Disord 1996;11 (Suppl 1):139.

29. Rascol O, Brooks DJ, Korczyn AD, et al. A five-year study of the incidence of dyskinesia in patients with early Parkinson's disease who were treated with ropinirole or levodopa. N Engl J Med 2000;342:1484-1491.

30. Whone AL, Remy P, Davis MR, et al. The REAL-PET study: slower progression in early Parkinson's disease treated with ropinirole compared with l-dopa. Neurology 2002;58 (suppl 3):A82-A83.

31. Ling ZD, Robie HC, Tong CW, Carvey PM. Both the antioxidant and D3 agonist actions of pramipexole mediate its neuroprotective actions in mesencephalic cultures. J Pharmacol Exp Ther 1999;289:202-210.

32. Shannon KM, Bennett JP Jr, Friedman JH. Efficacy of pramipexole, a novel dopamine agonist, as monotherapy in mild to moderate Parkinson's disease. The Pramipexole Study Group. Neurology 1997;49:724-728.

33. Lieberman A, Ranhosky A, Korts D. Clinical evaluation of pramipexole in advanced Parkinson's disease: results of a double-blind, placebo-controlled, parallel-group study. Neurology 1997;49:162-168.

34. Weiner WJ, Factor SA, Jankovic J, et al. The long term safety and efficacy of pramipexole in advanced Parkinson's disease. Parkinsonism Rel Disord 2001;7:115-120.

35. Parkinson Study Group. Pramipexole versus levodopa as initial treatment for Parkinson's disease: a randomized controlled trial. JAMA 2000;284:1931-1938.

36. Parkinson Study Group. Dopamine transporter brain imaging to assess the effects of pramipexole versus levodopa on Parkinson's disease progression. JAMA 2002;287: 1653-1661.

37. Pontiroli AE. Inhibition of basal and metoclopramide-induced prolactin release by cabergoline, an extremely long-acting dopaminergic drug. J Clin Endocrinol Metab 1987;65:1057-1059.

38. Ferrari C, Barbieri C, Caldara R, et al. Long-lasting prolactin lowering effect of cabergoline, a new dopamine agonist, in hyperprolactinemic patients. J Clin Endocrinol Met 1986;63:941-945.

39. Ahlskog JE, Muenter MD, Maraganore DM, Matsumoto JY, Lieberman A. Fluctuating Parkinson's disease:treatment with long-acting dopamine agonist cabergoline. Arch Neurol 1994;51:1236-1241.

40. Hutton JT, Morris JL, Brewer MA. Controlled study of the antiparkinsonian activity and tolerability of cabergoline. Neurology 1993;43:613-616.

41. Gopinathan G, Teravainen H, Dambrosia JM. Lisuride in parkinsonism. Neurology 1981;31:371-376.

42. Obeso JA, Luquin MR, Martinez J. Intravenous lisuride corrects oscillations of motor performance in Parkinson's disease. Ann Neurol 1986;19:31-35.

43. Obeso JA, Luquin MR, Vaamonde J, et al. Subcutaneous administration of lisuride in the treatment of complex motor fluctuations in Parkinson's disease. J Neurol Trans 1988;27:S17-25.

44. Barker R, Duncan J, Lees AJ. Subcutaneous apomorphine as a diagnostic test for dopaminergic responsiveness in parkinsonian syndromes. Lancet 1989;1:675.

45. Gylys JA, Wright RN, Nicolosi WD, Buyinski JP, Crenshaw RR. BMY-25801, an antiemetic agent free of D2-dopamine receptor antagonist properties. J Pharmacol Exp Ther 1988;244:830-7.

46. Goiny M, Unvan-Moberg K. Effects of dopamine receptor antagonists on gastrin and vomiting responses to apomorphine. Naunyn-Schmiedeberg's Arch Pharmacol 1987;336:16-19.

47. Montastruc JL, Rascol O, Senard JM, Rascol A. A randomised controlled study comparing bromocriptine to which levodopa was later added, with levodopa alone in previously untreated patients with Parkinson's disease: a five year follow up. Jour Neurol Neurosurg Psych 1994;57:1034-1038.

48. Hely MA, Morris JGL, Reid WGJ, O'Sullivan DJ, Williamson PM. The Sydney Multicentre Study of Parkinson's Disease: a randomized, prospective five year study comparing low-dose bromocriptine with low dose levodopa-carbidopa. Jour Neurol Neurosurg Psych 1994;57:903-910.

49. Rinne UK. Early dopamine agonist therapy in Parkinson's disease. Movement Disorders 1989;4:S86-94.

50. Frucht S, Rogers JD, Greene PE, et al. Falling asleep at the wheel: motor vehicle mishaps in persons taking pramipexole and ropinirole. Neurology 1999;52:1908-1910.

51. Hobson DE, Lang AE, Martin WR, Razmy A, Rivest J, Fleming J. Excessive daytime sleepiness and sudden onset sleep in Parkinson's disease; a survey by the Canadian Movement Disorders Group. JAMA 2002;287:455-463.

52. Ondo WG, Dat Wong K, Kahn H, Atassi F, Kwak C, Jankovic J. Daytime sleepiness and other sleep disorders in Parkinson's disease. Neurology 2001;57:1392-1396.

53. Axelrod J, Senoh S, Witkop B. O-methylation of catechol amines in vivo. J Biol Chem 1958;233:697-701.

54. Guldberg HC, Marsden CA. Catechol-O-methyl transferase: pharmacological aspects and physiological role. Pharmacol Rev 1975;27:135-206.

55. Nissenen E, Tuominen R, Perhoniemi V, Kaakkola S. Catechol-O-methyltransferase activity in human and rat small intestine. Life Sci 1988;42:2609-2614.

56. Kastner A, Anglade P, Bounaix C, Damier P, Javoy-Agid F et al. Immunohistochemical study of catechol-O-methyltransferase in the human mesostriatal system. Neuroscience 1994;62:449-457.

57. Reeches A, Meilke LR, Fahn S. 3-O-methyldopa inhibits rotations induced by levodopa in rats after unilateral destruction of the nigrostriatal pathway. Neurology 1982;32:887-888.

58. Nutt JG, Woodward WR, Gancher ST, Merrick D. 3-O-methyldopa and the response to levodopa in Parkinson's disease. Ann Neurol 1987;21:584-588.

59. Kaakkola S, Wurtman RJ. Effects of catechol-O-methyltransferase inhibitors and L-3,4-dihydroxyphenylalanine with or without carbidopa on extracellular dopamine in rat striatum. J Neurochem 1993;60:137-144.

60. Kaakkola S, Teravainen H, Ahtila S, Rita H, Gordin A. Effect of entacapone, a COMT inhibitor, on clinical disability and levodopa metabolism in parkinsonism patients. Neurology 1994;44:77-80.

61. Keranen T, Gordin A, Harjola VP, Karlsson M, Lorpela K. The effect of catechol-O-methyl transferase inhibition by entacapone on the pharmacokinetics and metabolism of levodopa in healthy volunteers. Clin Neuropharm 1993;16:145-156.

62. Rinne UK, Gordin A, Teravainen H. COMT inhibition with entacapone in the treatment of Parkinson's diseaes. Ann Neurol 1999;80:491-494.

63. Parkinson Study Group. Entacapone improves motor fluctuation in levodopa-treated Parkinson's disease patients. Ann Neurol 1997;42:747-755.

64. Rinne UK, Larsen JP, Siden A, Worm-Petersen J. Entacapone enhances the response to levodopa in parkinsonian patiens with motor fluctuations. Nomecomt Study Group. Neurology 1998;51:1309-1314.

64b. Larsen JP and the NOMESAFE study group. Poster, ICPDMD, 2001.

65. Hubble JP, Guarnieri M, Olanow CW. Effects of entacapone in Parkinson's disease patients without end of dose wearing off. Neurology 2003 (In Press).

66. Dingemanse J, Jorga K, Zurcher G, Schmitt M, Sedek G et al. Pharmokinetic-pharmacodynamic interaction between the COMT inhibitor tolcapone and single-dose levodopa. Br J Clin Pharmacol 1995;40:253-262.

67. Waters CH, Kurth M, Bailey P, et al. Tolcapone in stable Parkinson's disease: efficacy and safety of long term treatment. The Tolcapone Stable Study Group. Neurology 1997;49:665-671.

68. Rajput AH, Martin W, Saint-Hilaire MH, Dorflinger E, Pedder S. Tolcapone improves motor function in parkinsonian patients with the "wearing-off" phenomenon: a double-blind, placebo-controlled, multicenter trial. Neurology 1997;49:1066-1071.

69. Adler CH, Singer C, O'Brien C et al for the Tolcapone Study Group. Randomized, placebo-controlled study of tolcapone in patients with fluctuating Parkinson's disease treated with levodopa/carbidopa. Arch Neurol 1998;55:1089-1095.

70. Assal F, Spahr L, Hadengue A et al. Tolcapone and fulminant hepatitis. Lancet 1998;352:958.

71. Laine K, Anttila M, Heinonen E, et al. Lack of adverse interactions between concomitantly administered selegiline and citalopram. Clinical Neuropharmacology 1997;20:419-433.

72. Golbe LI. Long term efficacy and safety of deprenyl in advanced Parkinson's disease. Neurology 1989;39:1109-1111.

73. Birkmayer W, Riederer P, Youdim MBH et al. The potentiation of the anti-akinetic effect after L-dopa treatment by an inhibitor of MAO-B, Deprenil. J Neural Transm 1975;36:303-326.

74. Bodner RA, Lynch T, Lewis L, Kahn D. Serotonin syndrome. Neurology 1995;45:219-23.

75. Waters, C. Fluoxetine and selegiline-lack of significant interaction. Canadian Journal of Neurological Sciences 1994;21:259-261.

76. Parkinson Study Group. Effects of tocopherol and deprenyl on the progression of disability in early Parkinson's disease. N Engl J Med 1993;328:176-183.

77. Heikila RE, Manzino L, Cabbat FS, et al. Protection against the dopaminergic neurotoxicity of 1-methyl-4-phenyl-1,2,5,6-tetrahydropyridine by monoamine oxidase inhibitors. Nature 1984;311:467-469.

78. Parkinson Study Group. Effects of tocopherol and deprenyl on the progression of diability in early Parkinson's disease. N Engl J Med 1993;328:176-183.

78b. Parkinson Study Group. A controlled trial of rasagiline in early Parkinson disease: the TEMPO study. Arch Neurol 2002;59:1937-1943.

78c. Rabey JM, Sagi I, Huberman M, et al. Rasagiline mesylate, a new MAO-B inhibitor for the treatment of Parkinson's disease: a double-blind study as adjunctive therapy to levodopa. Clin Neuropharm 2000;23:324-330.

79. Jabbari B, Scherokman B, Gunderson CH et al. Treatment of movement disorders with trihexyphenidyl. Mov Disord 1989;4:202-212.

80. Butzer JF, Silver DE, Sahs AL. Amantadine in Parkinson's disease: a double-blind placebo-controlled cross-over study with long term follow-up. Neurology 1975;25:603-606.

81. Factor SA, Molho ES, Brown DL. Acute delirium after withdrawal of amantadine in Parkinson's disease. Neurology 1998;50:1456-1458.

82. Metman LV, DelDotto P, van DenMunckhof P et al. Amantadine as treatment for dyskinesias and motor fluctuations in Parkinson's disease. Neurology 1998;50:1323-1326.

83. Metman LV, DelDotto P, LePoole K et al. Amantadine for levodopa-induced dyskinesias. A 1-year follow-up study. Arch Neurol 1999;56:1383-1386.

84. Gerlak RP, Clark R, Stump JM et al. Amantadine-dopamine interaction. Science 1970;169:203-204.

Chapter 7 references

1. Pearce RK, Banerji T, Jenner P, Marsden CD. De novo administration of ropinirole and bromocriptine induces less dyskinesia than levodopa in MPTP-treated marmosets. Mov Disord 1998;13:234-241.

2. Montastruc JL, Rascol O, Senard JM, Rascol A. A randomised controlled study comparing bromocriptine to which levodopa was later added, with levodopa alone in previously untreated patients with Parkinson's disease: a five year follow up. J Neurol Neurosurg Psychiatry 1994;57:1034-1038.

3. Hely MA, Morris JGL, Reid WGJ, O'Sullivan DJ, Williamson PM. The Sydney Multicentre Study of Parkinson's disease: a randomized, prospective five year study comparing low dose bromocriptine with low dose levodopa-carbidopa. J Neurol Neurosurg Psychiatry 1994;57:903-910.

4. Rascol O, on behalf of the 056 Study Group. Ropinirole reduces the risk of dyskinesia when used in early PD. Parkinsonism Rel Disord 1999;5:S83-84.

5. Block G, Liss C, Reines S, Irr J, Nibbelink D, The CR First Study Group. Comparison of immediate-release and controlled release carbidopa/levodopa in Parkinson's disease. A multicenter 5-year study. Eur Neurol 1997;37:23-27.

6. Carter JH, Nutt JG, Woodward WR, Hatcher LF, Trotman TL. Amount and distribution of dietary protein affects clinical response to levodopa in Parkinson's disease. Neurology 1989;39:552-556.

7. Kurth MC, Tetrud JW, Irwin I, Lynes WH, Langston JW. Oral levodopa/carbidopa solution versus tablets in Parkinson's disease patients with severe fluctuations: a pilot study. Neurology 1993;43:1036-1039.

8. Metman LV, DelDotto P, van DenMunckhof P et al. Amantadine as treatment for dyskinesias and motor fluctuations in Parkinson's disease. Neurology 1998;50:1323-1326.

9. Lieberman A, Dziatolowski M, Kupersmith M, Serby M, Goodgold A, Korein J, Goldstein M. Dementia in Parkinson's disease. Ann Neurol 1979;6:355-359.

10. Baldessarini RJ, Frankenburg FR. Drug therapy: clozapine-a novel antipsychotic agent. N Engl J Med 1991;324:746-756.

11. Menza MM, Palermo B, Mark M. Quetiapine as an alternativde to clozapine in the treatment of dopamimetic psychosis in patients with Parkinson's disease. Ann Clin Psychiatry 1999;11:141-144.

12. Fernandez HH, Friedman JH, Jacques C, Rosenfield M. Quetiapine for the treatment of drug-induced psychosis in Parkinson's disease. Mov Disord 1999;14:484-487.

Chapter 8 references

1. Cummings JL. Depression and Parkinson's disease: a review. Am J Psychiatry 1992;149:443-454.

2. Ehmann TS, Beninger RJ, Gawal MJ, Riopelle RJ. Depressive symptoms in Parkinson's disease: a comparison with disabled control subjects. J Geriatr Psychiatry Neurol 1990;2:3-9.

3. Starkstein SE, Preziosi TJ, Bolduc PL, Robinson RG. Depression in Parkinson's disease. J Nerv Ment Dis 1990;178:27-31.

4. Gotham AM, Brown RG, Marsden CD. Depression in Parkinson's disease: a quantitative and qualitative analysis. J Neurol Neurosurg Psychiatry 1986;49:381-389.

5. Celesia GC, Wanamaker WM. Psychiatric disturbances in Parkinson's disease. Dis Nerv Syst 1972;33:577-583.

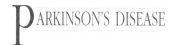

6. Mayeux R, Stern Y, Williams JBW, Cote L, Frantz A, Dyrenfurth I. Clinical and biochemical features of depression in Parkinson's disease. Am J Psychiatry 1986;143:756-759.

7. Mayeux R, Stern Y, Sano M, Williams JB, Cote LJ. The relationship of serotonin to depression in Parkinson's disease. Mov Disord 1988;3:237-244.

8. Andersen J, Aabro E, Gulmann N, Hjelmsted A, Pedersen HE. Anti-depressive treatment in Parkinson's disease: a controlled trial of the effect of nortriptyline in patients with Parkinson's disease treated with L-dopa. Acta Neurol Scan 1980;52:210-219.

9. Laitenen L. Desipramine in treatment of Parkinson's disease. Acta Neurol Scand 1969;45:109-113.

10. Goetz CG, Tanner CM, Klawans HL. Bupropion in Parkinson's disease. Neurology 1984;34:1092-1094.

11. Jansen-Steur ENH. Increase of Parkinson disability after fluoxetine medication. Neurology 1993;43:211-213.

12. Jimenez-Jimenez FJ, Tejeiro J, Martinez-Junquera G, Cabrera-Valdivia F, Alarcon J, et al. Parkinsonism exacerbated by paroxetine. Neurology 1994;44:2406.

13. Hauser RA, Zesiewicz TA. Sertraline for the treatment of depression in Parkinson's disease. Mov Disord 1997;12:756-759.

14. Sternbach H. The serotonin syndrome. Am J Psychiatry 1991;148:705-713.

15. Nirenberg DW, Semprebon M. The central nervous system serotonin syndrome. Clin Pharmacol Ther 1993;84-88.

16. Tackley RM, Tregaskis B. Fatal disseminated intravascular coagulation following a monoamine oxidase inhibitor/tricyclic interaction. Anaesthesia 1987;42:760-763.

17. Corkeron MA. Serotonin syndrome - a potentially fatal complication of antidepressant therapy. Med J Austral 1995;163:481-482.

18. Waters CH. Fluoxetine and selegiline - lack of significant interaction. Can J Neurol 1994;21:259-261.

19. Richard IH, Kurlan R, Tanner C et al. Serotonin syndrome and the combined use of deprenyl and an antidepressant in Parkinson's disease. Parkinson Study Group. Neurology 1997;48:1070-1077.

20. Hickler RB, Thompson GR, Fox LM, Hamlin JT. Successful treatment of orthostatic hypotension with 9-alpha-fluorohydrocortisone. N Engl J Med 1959;261:788-791.

21. Kaufman H, Brannan T, Krakoff L, Yahr MD, Mandeli J. Treatment of orthostatic hypotension due to autonomic failure with a peripheral alpha-adrenergic agonist (midodrine). Neurology 1988;38:951-956.

22. Davies B, Bannister R, Sever P. Pressor amines and monoamineoxidase inhibitors for treatment of postural hypotension in autonomic failure: limitations and hazards. Lancet 1978;1:172-175.

23. McTavish D, Goa KL. Midodrine: a review of its pharmacological properties and therapeutic use in orthostatic hypotension and secondary hypotensive disorders. Drugs 1989;38:757-777.

24. Pittner H, Stormann H, Enzenhofer R. Pharmacodynamic actions of midodrine, a new alpha-adrenergic stimulating agent, and its main metabolite, ST 1059. Arzneim Forsch 1976;26:2145-2154.

25. Zachariah PK, Bloedow DC, Moyer TP, Sheps SG, Schirger A, et al. Pharmacodynamics of midodrine, an antihypotensive agent. Clin Pharmacol Ther 1986;39:586-591.

26. Jankovic J, Gilden JL, Hiner BC, Kaufman H, Brown DC. Neurogenic orthostatic hypotension: a double-blind placebo-controlled study with midodrine. Am J Med 1993;95:38-48.

27. Jost WH, Schimrigk K. Constipation in Parkinson's disease. Klinische Wochenschrift 1991;69:906-909.

28. Edwards LL, Quigley EMM, Harned RK, Hofman R, Pfeiffer R. Characterization of swallowing and defecation in Parkinson's disease. Am J Gastroenterol 1994;89:15-25.

29. Ashraf W, Pfeiffer R, Quigely EMM. Anorectal manometer in the assessment of anorectal function in Parkinson's disease: a comparison with chronic idiopathic constipation. Mov Disord 1994;9:655-663.

30. Mathers SE, Kempster PA, Law PJ, et al. Anal sphincter dysfunction in Parkinson's disease. Arch Neurol 1989;46:1061-1064.

31. Oyanagi K, Wakabayashi K, Ohama E, Takeda S, Horikawa Y, Morita T, Ikuta F. Lewy bodies in the lower sacral parasympathetic neurons of a patient with Parkinson's disease. Acta Neuropathol 1990;80:558-559.

32. Mathers SE, Kempster PA, Swash M, Lees AJ. Constipation and paradoxical puborectalis contraction in anismus and Parkinson's disease: a dystonic phenomenon? J Neurol Neurosurg Psych 1988;51:1503-1507.

33. Edwards LL, Pfeiffer RF, Quigley EMM, Hofman R, Balluff M. Gastrointestinal symptoms in Parkinson's disease. Movement Disorders 1991;6:151-156.

34. Edwards LL, Quigley EMM, Pfeiffer RF. Gastrointestinal dysfunction in Parkinson's disease: frequency and pathophysiology. Neurology 1992;42:726-732.

35. Bird MR, Woodward MC, Gibson EM, Phyland DJ, Fonda D. Asymptomatic swallowing disorders in elderly patients with Parkinson's disease: a description of findings on clinical examination and videofluoroscopy in sixteen patients. Age and Ageing 1994;23:251-254.

36. Qualman SJ, Haupt HM, Yang P, Hamilton SR. Esophageal Lewy bodies associated with ganglion cell loss in achalasia. Similarity to Parkinson's disease. Gastroenterology 1984;87:848-856.

37. Wang SJ, Chia LG, Hsu CY, Lin WY, Kao CH, Yeh SH. Dysphagia in Parkinson's disease. Assessment by solid phase radionuclide scintigraphy. Clin Nuc Med 1994;19:405-407.

38. Wintzen AR, Badrising UA, Roos RA, Vielvoye J, Liauw L, Pauwels EK. Dysphagia in ambulant patients with Parkinson's disease: common, not dangerous. Can J Neur Sci 1994;212:53-56.

39. Bushman M, Dobmeyer SM, Leeker L, Perlmutter JS. Swallowing abnormalities and their responses to treatment in Parkinson's disease. Neurology 1989;39:1309-1314.

40. Khan Z, Starer P, Bhola A. Urinary incontinence in female Parkinson's disease patients. Urology 1989;33:486-489.

41. Suchowersky O, Furtado S, Rohs G. Beneficial effect of intranasal desmopressin for nocturnal polyuria in Parkinson's disease. Mov Disord1995;10:337-340.

42. Lipe, H, Longstreth WT, Bird TD, Linde M. Sexual function in married men with Parkinson's disease compared to married men with arthritis. Neurology 1990;40:1347-1349.

43. Rosen RC, Kostis JB, Jekelis AW. Beta-blocker effects on sexual function in normal males. Arch Sex Behavior 1988;17:241-55.

44. Smith PJ, Talbert RL. Sexual dysfunction with antihypertensive and antipsychotic agents. Clinical Pharmacy 1986;5:373-84.

45. Zesiewicz TA, Helal M, Hauser RA. Sildenafil Citrate (Viagra) for the treatment of erectile dysfunction in men with Parkinson's disease. Mov Disord 2000;15:305-308.

46. Hauser RA, Wahba MN, Zesiewicz TA, Anderson WM. Modafinil treatment of pramipexole associated somnolence. Mov Disord 2000;15:1269-1271.

47. Nieves AV, Land AE. Treatment of excessive daytime sleepiness in patients with Parkinson's disease with modafinil. Clin Neuropharm 2002;25:11-114.

48. Bilowit DS. Establishing physical objectives in the rehabilitation of patients with Parkinson's disease (gymnasium activities). Phys Ther Rev 1956;36:176-178.

49. Hurwitz A. The benefit of a home exercise regimen for ambulatory Parkinson's disease patients. J Neurosci Nursing 1989;21:180-184.

50. Comella CL, Stebbins GT, Brown-Toms BA, Goetz C. Physical therapy and Parkinson's disease: a controlled clinical trial. Neurology 1994;44:376-378.

Chapter 9 references

1. Koller WC, Pahwa R, Lyons KE, Albanese A. Surgical treatment of Parkinson's disease. J Neurol Sci. 1999;167:1-10.

2. Spiegel EA, Wycis HT, Marks M, al. e. Stereotaxic apparatus for operations on the human brain. Science. 1947;106:349-350

3. Hassler R, Riechert T. Indikationen and Lokalisationsmethode der gerielten Hirnoperationen. Nervenarzt. 1954;25:441-447.

4. Svennilson E, Torvik A, Lowe R, al. e. Treatment of parkinsonism by stereotactic thermolesions in the pallidal region. A clinical evaluation of 81 cases. Acta Psychiatr Neurol Scand. 1960;35:358-377

5. Benabid AL, Pollak P, Louveau A et al. Combined (thalamotomy and stimulation) stereotactic surgery of the VIM thalamic nucleus for bilateral Parkinson disease. Appl Neurophysiol. 1987;50:344-346

6. Kelly PJ, Gillingham FJ. The long term results of stereotaxic surgery and L-dopa therapy in patients with Parkinson's disease. A 10-year follow-up study. J Neurosurg. 1980;53:332-337

7. Nagaseki Y, Shibazaki T, Hirai T et al. Long term follow-up results of selective VIM-thalamotomy. J Neurosurg. 1986;65:296-302

8. Jankovic J, Cardoso F, Grossman RG, Hamilton WJ. Outcome after stereotactic thalamotomy for parkinsonian, essential, and other types of tremor [see comments]. Neurosurgery. 1995;37:680-686; discussion 686-687

9. Diederich N, Goetz CG, Stebbins GT et al. Blinded evaluation confirms long term asymmetric effect of unilateral thalamotomy or subthalamotomy on tremor in Parkinson's disease. Neurology. 1992;42:1311-1314

10. Blond S, Caparros-Lefebvre D, Parker F et al. Control of tremor and involuntary movement disorders by chronic stereotactic stimulation of the ventral intermediate thalamic nucleus. J Neurosurg. 1992;77:62-68

11. Speelman JD, Bosch DA. [Continuous electric thalamus stimulation for the treatment of tremor resistant to pharmacotherapy]. Ned Tijdschr Geneeskd. 1995;139:926-930

12. Alesch F, Pinter MM, Helscher RJ et al. Stimulation of the ventral intermediate thalamic nucleus in tremor dominated Parkinson's disease and essential tremor. Acta Neurochir. 1995;136:75-81

13. Benabid AL, Pollak P, Gao D et al. Chronic electrical stimulation of the ventralis intermedius nucleus of the thalamus as a treatment of movement disorders [see comments]. J Neurosurg. 1996;84:203-214

14. Koller W, Pahwa R, Busenbark K et al. High-frequency unilateral thalamic stimulation in the treatment of essential and parkinsonian tremor. Ann Neurol. 1997;42:292-299

15. Ondo W, Jankovic J, Schwartz K et al. Unilateral thalamic deep brain stimulation for refractory essential tremor and Parkinson's disease tremor. Neurology. 1998;51:1063-1069

16. Limousin P, Speelman JD, Gielen F, Janssens M. Multicentre European study of thalamic stimulation in parkinsonian and essential tremor. J Neurol Neurosurg Psychiatry. 1999;66:289-296

17. Pollak P, Benabid AL, Limousin P, Benazzouz A. Chronic intracerebral stimulation in Parkinson's disease. Adv Neurol. 1997;74:213-220

18. Lyons KE, Koller WC, Wilkinson SB, Pahwa R. Long term safety and efficacy of unilateral deep brain stimulation of the thalamus for parkinsonian tremor. J Neurol Neurosurg Psychiatry. 2001;71:682-684

19. Alkhani A, Lozano AM. Pallidotomy for parkinson disease: a review of contemporary literature. J Neurosurg. 2001;94:43-49.

20. Lang AE, Lozano AM, Montgomery E et al. Posteroventral medial pallidotomy in advanced Parkinson's disease [see comments]. N Engl J Med. 1997;337:1036-1042

21. Pal PK, Samii A, Kishore A et al. Long term outcome of unilateral pallidotomy: follow up of 15 patients for 3 years. J Neurol Neurosurg Psychiatry. 2000;69:337-344.

22. Hariz MI, Bergenheim AT. A 10-year follow-up review of patients who underwent Leksell's posteroventral pallidotomy for Parkinson disease. J Neurosurg. 2001;94:552-558.

23. Kumar R, Lozano AM, Montgomery E, Lang AE. Pallidotomy and deep brain stimulation of the pallidum and subthalamic nucleus in advanced Parkinson's disease. Mov Disord. 1998;13:73-82

24. Deep-brain stimulation of the subthalamic nucleus or the pars interna of the globus pallidus in Parkinson's disease. N Engl J Med. 2001;345:956-963.

25. Ghika J, Villemure JG, Fankhauser H et al. Efficiency and safety of bilateral contemporaneous pallidal stimulation (deep brain stimulation) in levodopa-responsive patients with Parkinson's disease with severe motor fluctuations: a 2-year follow-up review. J Neurosurg. 1998;89:713-718

26. Volkmann J, Sturm V, Weiss P et al. Bilateral high-frequency stimulation of the internal globus pallidus in advanced Parkinson's disease. Ann Neurol. 1998;44:953-961

27. Durif F, Lemaire JJ, Debilly B, Dordain G. Long term follow-up of globus pallidus chronic stimulation in advanced Parkinson's disease. Mov Disord. 2002;17:803-807

28. Abosch A, Lang AE, Hutchinson WD, Lozano AM. Subthalamic Deep Brain Stimulation for Parkinson's Disease. In: Tarsy D, Vitek JL, Lozano AM, eds. Surgical Treatment of Parkinson's Disease and Other Movement Disorders. Totowa, New Jersey: Humana Press, 2002:175-189

29. Kumar R, Lozano AM, Kim YJ et al. Double-blind evaluation of subthalamic nucleus deep brain stimulation in advanced Parkinson's disease. Neurology. 1998;51:850-855.

30. Limousin P, Krack P, Pollak P et al. Electrical stimulation of the subthalamic nucleus in advanced Parkinson's disease. N Engl J Med. 1998;339:1105-1111

31. Krack P, Pollak P, Limousin P et al. Subthalamic nucleus or internal pallidal stimulation in young onset Parkinson's disease. Brain. 1998;121:451-457

32. Benabid AL, Krack PP, Benazzouz A et al. Deep brain stimulation of the subthalamic nucleus for Parkinson's disease: methodologic aspects and clinical criteria. Neurology. 2000;55:S40-44.

33. Rodriguez-Oroz MC, Gorospe A, Guridi J et al. Bilateral deep brain stimulation of the subthalamic nucleus in Parkinson's disease. Neurology. 2000;55:S45-51.

34. Gill SS, Patel NK, Heywood P. Subthalamotomy for Parkinson's Disease. In: Tarsy D, Vitek J, Lozano AM, eds. Surgical Treatment of Parkinson's Disease and Other Movement Disorders. Totowa: Humana Press, 2002:145-152

35. Burchiel KJ, Anderson VC, Favre J, Hammerstad JP. Comparison of pallidal and subthalamic nucleus deep brain stimulation for advanced Parkinson's disease: results of a randomized, blinded pilot study. Neurosurgery. 1999;45:1375-1382; discussion 1382-1374.

36. Volkmann J, Allert N, Voges J et al. Safety and efficacy of pallidal or subthalamic nucleus stimulation in advanced PD. Neurology. 2001;56:548-551

37. Pollak P, Fraix V, Krack P et al. Treatment results: Parkinson's disease. Mov Disord. 2002;17:S75-83.

38. Oh MY, Abosch A, Kim SH et al. Long term hardware-related complications of deep brain stimulation. Neurosurgery. 2002;50:1268-1274; discussion 1274-1266

39. Perlow M, Freed WJ, Hoffer BJ, et al. Brain grafts reduce motor abnormalities produced by destruction of nigro-striatal dopamine system. Science 1979;204:643-647.

40. Bjorklund A, Kromer LF, Stenevi U. Cholinergic reinnervation of the rat hippocampus by septal implants is stimulated by perforant path lesion. Brain Res 1979;173:57-64.

41. Bjorklund A, Stenevi U, Schmidt RH, et al. Intracerebral grafting of neuronal cell suspensions. I. Introduction and general methods of preparation. Acta Physiol Scand 1983;522:9-18.

42. Mahalick TJ, Finger TE, Stromberg I, et al. Substantia nigra transplants into denervated striatum of the rat: Ultrastructure of graft-host interconnections. J Comp Neurol 1985;240:60-70.

43. Wuerthele SM, Freed WJ, Olson L, et al. Effects of dopamine agonists and antagonists on the electrical activity of substantia nigra neurons tranpslanted into the lateral ventricle of the rat. Exp Brain Res 1981;44:1-10.

44. Schmidt RH, Ingvar M, Lindvall O, et al. Functional activity of substantia nigra grafts reinnervating the striatum: neurotransmitter metabolism and [14C]-2deoxy-D-glucose autoradiography. J Neurochem 1982;38:737-748.

45. Brundin P, Bjorklund A. Survival, growth and function of dopaminergic neurons grafted to the brain. Prog Brain Res 1987;71:293-308.

46. Sladek JR, Collier TC, Haber SN, et al. Survival and growth of fetal catecholamine neurons transplanted into the primate brain. Brain Res Bull 1986;17:809-818.

47. Bakay RAE, Barrow DL, Fiandca MS, et al. Biochemical and behavioral correction of MPTP-like syndrome by fetal transplantation. Ann NY Acad Sci 1987;495:623-640.

48. Sladek JR, Redmond DE, Collier TC, et al. Fetal dopamine neural grafts: extended reversal of methylphenyltetrahydropyridine-induced parkinsonism in primates. Prog Brain Res 1988;78:497-506.

49. Fine A, Hunt SB, Oertel WH, et al. Transplantation of embryonic dopaminergic neurons to the corpus striatum of marmosets rendered parkinsonian by 1-methyl-4-phenyl-1,2,3,6-tetrahydropyridine. Prog Brain Res 1988;78:479-490.

50. Bohn MC, Cupit L, Marciano F, et al. Adrenal medulla autografts into the basal ganglia of cebus monkeys: injury-induced regeneration. Exp Neurol 1988;102:76-91.

51. Backlund EO, Granberg PO, Hamerger B, et al. Transplantation of adrenal medullary tissue to striatum in parkinsonism. First clinical trials. J Neurosurg 1985;62:169-173.

52. Lindvall O, Backlund EO, Farde L, et al. Transplantation in Parkinson's disease: two cases of adrenal medullary grafts to the putamen. Ann Neurol 1987;22:457-468.

53. Madrazo I, Drucker-Colin R, Diaz V, et al. Open microsurgical autograft of adrenal medulla to right caudate nucleus in two patients with intractable Parkinson's disease. NEJM 1987;316:831-834.

54. Lieberman A, Ransohoff J, Berczeller P, et al. Neural and adrenal medullary transplants as a treatment for Parkinson's disease and other neurodegenerative disorders. Trends Clin Neurol 1988;4:1-15.

55. Penn RD, Goetz CG, Tanner CM, et al. The adrenal medullary transplant operation for Parkinson's disease: clinical observations in five patients. Neurosurgery 1988;22:999-1004.

56. Allen GS, Burns RS, Tulipan NB, et al. Adrenal medullary transplantation to the caudate nucleus in Parkinson's disease. Initial clinical results in 18 patients. Arch Neurol 1989; 46:487-491.

57. Goetz CG, Olanow CW, Koller WC, et al. Multicenter study of autologous adrenal medullary transplantation to the corpus striatum in patients with advanced Parkinson's disease. NEJM 1989;320:337-341.

58. Jankovic J. Grossman R, Goodman C, et al. Clinical, biochemical, and neuropathologic findings following transplantation of adrenal medulla to the caudate nucleus for treatment of Parkinson's disease. Neurology 1989;39:1227-1234.

59. Kelly PJ, Ahlskog JE, vanHeerden JA, et al. Adrenal medullary autograft transplantation into the striatum of patients with Parkinson's disease. Mayo Clin Proc 1989;64:282-290.

60. Ahlskog JE, Kelly PH, vanHeerden JA, et al. Adrenal medullary transplantation into the brain for treatment of Parkinson's disease: clinical outcome and neurochemical studies. Mayo Clin Proc 1990;65:305-328.

61. Apuzzo MLJ, Neal JH, Waters CH, et al. Utilization of unilateral and bilateral stereotactically placed adrenomedullary-striatal autografts in parkinsonian humans: rationale, techniques and observations. Neurosurgery 1990;26:746-757.

62. Koller WC, Waxman M, Morantz R. Adrenal neural transplants in Parkinson's disease. Adv Neurol 1990;53:559-565.

63. Olanow CW, Koller WC, Goetz CG, et al. Autologous transplantation of adrenal medulla in Parkinson's disease. Arch Neurol 1990;47:1286-1289.

64. Goetz CG, Stebbins GT, Klawans HL, et al. United Parkinson Foundation neurotransplantation registry on adrenal medullary transplant: presurgical, and 1-and 2-year follow-up. Neurology 1991;41:1719-1722.

65. Frank F, Sturiale C, Gaist C, et al. Adrenal medulla autograft in a human brain for Parkinson's disease. Acta Neurochir 1988;94:39.

66. Hurtig H, Joyce J, Sladek JR, et al. Post-mortem analysis of adrenal medulla-to-caudate autogaft in a patient with Parkinson's disease. Ann Neurol 1989;25:607-614.

67. Waters C, Itabashi HH, Apuzzo MLJ, et al. Adrenal to caudate transplantation-post mortem study. Mov Disord 1990;5:248-250.

68. Kordower JH, Cochran E, Penn R, et al. Putative chromaffin cell survival and enhanced host derived TH-fiber innervation following a functional adrenal medulla autogaft for Parkinson's disease. Ann Neurol 1991;29:405-412.

69. Lindvall O, Rechncrona S, Gustaavii N, et al. Fetal dopamine-rich mesencephalic grafts in Parkinson's disease. Lancet 1988;1483-1484.

70. Lindvall O, Rehncrona S, Brundin P, et al. Human fetal dopamine neurons grafted into the striatum in two patients with Parkinson's disease: a detailed account of methodology and 6 month follow-up. Arch Neurol 1989;46:615-631.

71. Lindvall O, Brundin P, Widner H, et al. Grafts of fetal dopamine neurons survive and improve motor function in Parkinson's disease. Science 1990;247:574-577.

72. Lindvall O, Widner H, Rehncrona S, et al. Transplantation of fetal dopamine neurons in Parkinson's disease: one-year clinical and neurophysiological observations in two patients with putaminal implants. Ann Neurol 1992;31:155-165.

73. Sawle GV, Bloomfield PM, Bjorklund A, et al. Transplantation of fetal dopamine neurons in Parkinson's disease: PET 18F-6- fluorodopa studies in two patients with putaminal implants. Ann Neurol 1992;31:166-173.

74. Freed CR, Breeze RE, Rosenberg NL, et al. Transplantation of human fetal dopamine cells for Parkinson's disease. Results at one year. Arch Neurol 1990;47:505-512.

75. Freed CR, Breeeze RE, Rosenberg NL, et al. Survival of implanted fetal dopamine cells and neurologic improvement 12 to 46 months after transplantation for Parkinson's disease. NEJM 1992;327:1549-1555.

76. Spencer DD, Robbins RJ, Naftolin F, et al. Unilateral transplantation of human fetal mesencephalic tissue into the caudate nucleus of patients with Parkinson's disease. NEJM 1992;327:1541-1548.

77. Widner H, Tetrud J, Rehncrona S, et al. Bilateral fetal mesencephalic grafting in two patients with parkinsonism induced by 1-methyl-4-phenyl-1,2,3,6-tetrahydropyridine (MPTP). NEJM 1992;327:1556-63.

78. Freed CR, Breeze RE, Rosenberg NL, et al. Transplantation of human fetal dopamine cells for Parkinson's disease: results at 1 year. Arch Neurol 1990;47:505-512.

79. Lindvall O, Brundin P, Widner H, et al. Grafts of fetal dopamine neurons survive and improve motor function in Parkinson's disease. Science 1990;247:574-577.

80. Freed CR, Breeze RE, Resenberg NL, et al. Fetal neural implants for Parkinson's disease: results at 15 months. In: Lindvall O, Bjorklund A, Winder H, et al. Intracerbral transplantation in movement disorders. Vol 4 of Restorative neurology. Amsterdam: Elsevier, 1991;69-77.

81. Freed CR, Breeze RE, Rosenberg NL, et al. Survival of implanted fetal dopamine cells and neurologic improvement 12 to 46 months after transplantation for Parkinson's disease. N Engl J Med 1992;327:1549-1555.

82. Breeze RE, Wells TH Jr, Freed CR. Implantation of fetal tissue for the management of Parkinson's disease: a technical note. Neurosurgery 1995;36:1044-1047.

83. Spencer DD, Robbins Rj, Naftolin F, et al. Unilateral transplantation of human fetal mesencephalic tissue into the caudate nucleus of patients with Parkinson's disease. N Engl J Med 1992;327:1541-1548.

84. Widner H, Tetrud J, Rehncrona S, et al. Bilateral fetal mesencephalic grafting in two patients with parkinsonism induced by 1-methyl-4-phenyl-1,2,3,6-tetrahydropyridine (MPTP). N Engl J Med 1992;327:1556-1563.

85. Lindvall O, Sawle G, Widner H, et al. Evidence for long term survival and function of dopaminergic grafts in progressive Parkinson's disease. Ann Neurol 1994;35:172-180.1995:1677-1687.

86. Freeman TB, Olanow CW, Hauser RA, et al. Bilateral fetal nigral transplantation into the postcommissural putamen in Parkinson's disease. Ann Neurol 1995;38:379-388.

87. Kordower JH, Freeman TB, Snow BJ, et al. Neuropathological evidence of graft survival and striatal reinnervation after the transplantation of fetal mesencephalic tissue in a patient with Parkinson's disease. N Engl J Med 1995;332:1118-11124.

88. Peschanski M, Deger G, N'Guyuen JP, et al. Bilateral motor improvement and alteration of L-dopa effect in two patients with Parkinson's disease following intrastriatal transplantation of foetal ventral mesencephalon. Brain 1994;17:487-499.

89. Defer GL, Geny C, Ricolfi F, et al. Long term outcome of uniliaterally transplanted parkinsonian patients. I. Clinical approach. Brain 1996;119:41-50.

90. Kopyov OV, Jacques D, Lieberman A, et al. Clinical study of fetal mesencephalic intracerebral transplants for the treatment of Parkinson's disease. Cell Transplant 1996;5:327-337.

91. Hauser RA, Freeman TB, Snow BJ, et al. Long term evaluation of bilateral fetal nigral transplantation in Parkinson's disease. Arch Neurol 1999;56:179-187.

92. Wenning GK, Odin P, Morrish P, et al. Short- and long term survival and function of unilateral intrastriatal dopaminergic grafts in Parkinson's disease. Ann Neurol 1997;42:95-107.

93. Piccini P, Brooks DJ, Bjorklund A, et al. Dopamine release from nigral transplants visualized in vivo in a Parkinson's patient. Nat Neurosci 1999;12:1137-1140.

94. Kordower JH, Freeman TB, Chen EY, et al. Fetal nigral grafts survive and mediate clinical benefit in a patient with Parkinson's disease. Mov Disord 1998;13:383-393.

95. Lindvall O, Widner H, Rehncrona S, et al. Transplantation of fetal dopamine neurons in Parkinson's disease: one-year clinical and neurophysiological observations in two patients with putaminal implants. Arch Neurol 1992;31:155-173.

96. Hallett M, Litvan I, and the Task Force on Surgery for Parkinson's dsease. Evaluation of surgery for Parkinson's disease. Neurology 1999;53:1910-1921.

97. Freeman RB, Willing A, Zigova T et al. Neural transplantation in Parkinson's disease. Adv Neurol 2001;86:435-445.

98. Kordower JH, Rosenstein JM, Collier TJ, et al. Functional fetal nigral grafts in a patient with Parkinson's disease: chemoanatomic, ultrastructural and metabolic studies. J Comp Neurol 1996;370:203-230.

99. Freeman TB, Vawter DE, Leaverton PE, et al. Use of placebo surgery in controlled trials of a cellular-based therapy for Parkinson's disease. N Engl J Med. 1999 Sep 23;341(13):988-92.

100. Freed CR, Greene PE, Breeze RE et al. Transplantation of embryonic dopamine neurons for severe Parkinson's disease. N Eng J Med 2001;344:710-19.

101. Ma Y, Feigin A, Dhawan V, et al. Dyskinesia after fetal cell transplantation for parkinsonism: a PET study. Ann Neurol 2002;52:628-634.

102. Olanow C. Transplantation for Parkinson's disease: Pros, cons, and where do we go from here? Mov Disord 2002;17:S15.

103. Schumacher JM, Ellias SA, Palmer EP, et al. Transplantation of embryonic porcine mesencephalic tissue in patients with PD. Neurology. 2000 Mar 14;54(5):1042-50.

104. Deacon T, Schumacher J, Dinsmore J, et al. Histological evidence of fetal pig neural cell survival after transplantation into a patient with Parkinson's disease. Nat Med. 1997 Mar;3(3):350-3.

105. Hauser RA, Watts RL, Freeman TB. A double-blind, randomized, controlled, multicenter clinical trial of the safety and efficacy of transplanted fetal porcine ventral mesencephalic cells versus imitation surgery in patients with Parkinson's disease. Mov Disord 2001;16:983-984.

107. Watts RL, Raiser C, Stover N, et al. Stereotaxic intrastriatal implantation of retinal pigment epithelial cells attached to microcarriers in advanced Parkinson disease patients: long term follow-up. Neurology 2002;58:A241.

108. Arenas E. Stem cells in the treatment of Parkinson's disease.Brain Res Bull. 2002 Apr;57(6):795-808.

109. Kordower JH, Emborg ME, Bloch J, et al. Neurodegeneration prevented by lentiviral vector delivery of GDNF in primate models of Parkinson's disease. Science 2000;290(5492):767-773.

110. Akerud P, Canals JM, Snyder EY, Arenas E. Neuroprotection through delivery of glial cell line-derived neurotrophic factor by neural stem cells in a mouse model of Parkinson's disease. J Neurosci. 2001 Oct 15;21(20):8108-18.

111. Gill S, Nikunj K, O'Sullivan K, et al. Intraparenchymal putaminal administration of glial-derived neurotrophic factor in treatment of advanced Parkinson's disease. Neurology 2002;58:A241.

Chapter 10 references

1. National Parkinson Foundation, Bob Hope Parkinson Research Center, 1501 N.W. 9th Avenue, Miami Fl 33136-1494, 1-800-327-4545. www.parkinson.org

2. The American Parkinson Disease Association, 1250 Hylan Boulevard, Suite 4B, Staten Island, NY 10305-1946, 1-800-223-2732; www.apdaparkinson.com

3. Parkinson's Disease Foundation, Inc. William Black Medical Building, Columbia-Presbyterian Medical Center, 710 West 168th Street, New York, NY, 10032-9982, 1-212-923-4700; 1-800-457-6676; www.info@pdf.org.

4. United Parkinson Foundation, 833 W Washington Boulevard, Chicago, IL, 60607, 1-312-733-1893.

5. International Tremor Foundation, 7046 W 105th St, Overland Park, KS 66212-1803, 1-913-341-3880, www.essentialtremor.org

6. American Academy of Neurology, 1080 Montreal Avenue, St. Paul, MN 55116, 1-651-695-1940, web@aan.com

7. We Move, 204 West 84th Street, NY, NY 10024, In the US, call 1-800-437-MOV2; outside the US, call 1-212-241-8567, e-mail: wemove@wemove.org

8. Society for Progressive Supranuclear Palsy, Suite 515, Woodholme Medical Building, 1838 Greene Tree Rd, Baltimore, MD 21208, 1-800-457-4777.

9. The Movement Disorder Society, 611 Wells Street, Milwaukee, WI, 53202; 1-414-276-2145.

ACKNOWLEDGMENTS

Figure 1-1. *Reprinted with kind permission from Duvoisin RC, Sage J. Parkinson's Disease: A Guide for Patient and Family. 4th Edition. Lippincot-Raven, 1996.*

Figure 1-2. *Reprinted with kind permission from Jankovic J, Tolosa E, Eds. Parkinson's Disease and Movement Disorders. Williams and Wilkins, 1993.*

Figure 1-5. *Reprinted with kind permission from Calne DB. Parkinsonism: Physiology, Pharmacology and Treatment. Edward Arnold, 1970.*

Figure 1-7. *Reprinted with kind permission from Calne DB. New England Journal of Medicine 1993;329:1022.*

Figure 1-8. *Reprinted with kind permission from Calne DB. New England Journal of Medicine 1993;329:1023.*

Figure 1-9. *Reprinted with kind permission from Calne DB. New England Journal of Medicine 1993;329:1023.*

Figure 2-2. *Reprinted with kind permission from Olanow CW. Ann Neurol 1992;32:S3.*

Figure 2-3. *Reprinted with kind permission from Olanow CW. Ann Neurol 1992;32:S3.*

Figure 2-4. *Reprinted with kind permission from Olanow CW. Ann Neurol 1992;32:S3.*

Figure 2-5. *Reprinted with kind permission from Cedarbaum JM, Grancher ST. Neurologic Clinics 1992;10:544.*

Figure 2-6. *Reprinted with kind permission from DiMonte D. Neurology 1991;41:39.*

Figure 6-1. *Reprinted with kind permission from Kaakkola S. Rinne UK, Gordin A. COMT Inhibition with Entacapone: a New Principle of Levodopa Extension. Koteva Oy, Tahitorni Oy; Finland 1996:13.*

Figure 6-2. *Reprinted with kind permission from Kaakkola S. Rinne UK, Gordin A. COMT Inhibition with Entacapone: a New Principle of Levodopa Extension. Koteva Oy, Tahitorni Oy; Finland 1996:14.*

Figure 6-3. *Reprinted with kind permission from Gordin A, Rinne UK. Rinne UK, Gordin A. COMT Inhibition with Entacapone: a New Principle of Levodopa Extension. Koteva Oy, Tahitorni Oy; Finland 1996:27.*

Figure 6-7. *Reprinted with kind permission from Appel SH, Ed. Current Neurology 1992;12:130.*

Figure 6-8. *Reprinted with kind permission from The Parkinson Study Group. New England Journal of Medicine 1993;328:178.*

We would like to thank Kelly E. Lyons, PhD for suggestions and editorial comments

COMPANION CD LEGENDS

Case 1. Mild Parkinson's Disease

This is a 58-year-old woman who first noticed tremor in the right hand one and a half years ago. She experienced progressive difficulty with fine coordinated movements in the right upper extremity and treatment was begun with a dopamine agonist nine months ago. Videotaped examination reveals mild right hand rest tremor. She has no postural or kinetic tremors. Extra-ocular movements are normal. Fine coordinated movements in the left upper extremity are normal. Fine coordinated movements in the right upper extremity are mildly decreased. Pronation-supination in the right hand is moderately decreased. Toe tapping is moderately decreased in both lower extremities, more on the right than the left. She is able to arise from a chair with arms crossed without difficulty. Gait consists of strides of normal length on a narrow base. Arm swing during ambulation is absent on the right and a mild rest tremor is observed in the right upper extremity. On pull test, she regains balance within two steps. This case demonstrates classic features of Parkinson's disease including asymmetric rest tremor and bradykinesia.

Case 2. Moderate Parkinson's Disease

This is a 42-year-old right handed woman who first noticed "dragging" of her left leg while running six years ago. Six months later, she developed tremor in the left hand. Over time she developed more stiffness and tightness in her left leg. She was initially treated with a dopamine agonist and amantadine was added later. Six months ago, levodopa/carbidopa and entacapone were added. Videotaped examination reveals a mild rest tremor in the left upper extremity. She also has slight kinetic and postural tremors in the left upper extremity. Blink rate is mild to moderately reduced. Fine coordinated movements are mildly reduced in the right upper extremity and moderately reduced in the left upper extremity. Decrementing (smaller amplitude with successive movements) is identified with hand opening and closing. Foot tapping is normal on the right and moderately reduced on the left. She is able to arise from a chair without difficulty. Gait consists of strides of normal length on a narrow base. Axial posture is slightly flexed. Arm swing during ambulation is absent on the left. On pull test, she regains balance with one step. This case demonstrates typical Parkinson's disease features including asymmetric rest tremor and bradykinesia. She is experiencing a stable response to medications but has residual signs and symptoms.

Case 3. Advanced Parkinson's Disease with Motor Fluctuations and Dyskinesia

This is a 62-year-old man who was diagnosed with Parkinson's Disease 12 years ago. He initially noticed tremor in the left arm and leg. He was treated with levodopa/carbidopa and trihexyphenidyl beginning 10 years ago. He developed wearing off motor fluctuations on levodopa/carbidopa beginning seven years ago. Dyskinesia emerged one year later. He is currently treated with levodopa/carbidopa 100/25 $1^1/_2$ tablet five times per day on an every

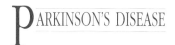

three hour schedule. He also takes trihexyphenidyl 2 mg. four times per day. He reports that he is OFF approximately 20% of the day and has dyskinesia approximately 10% of the day. Increasing levodopa/carbidopa increases dyskinesia and lowering levodopa/carbidopa increases OFF time.

A. Examination in the OFF state reveals a moderate decrease in blink rate and a mild decrease in facial expression. He has a moderate amplitude rest tremor in the left upper extremity and a mild rest tremor in the right upper extremity. With arms outstretched, he has a moderate postural tremor in the left upper extremity and a mild postural tremor in the right upper extremity. Fine coordinated movements are mildly reduced bilaterally. Foot tapping is slightly reduced on the right and mildly reduced on the left. He is able to arise from a chair with mild slowness. There is moderate start-hesitation. Gait consists of strides of slightly shortened length on a narrow base. He has en bloc turning with some tendency for freezing. Axial posture is mildly flexed. Arm swing is reduced bilaterally during ambulation. On pull test, he regains balance in three steps.

B. Examination while ON demonstrates resolution of tremor. He has moderate dyskinesia in the head and mild dyskinesia in the right hand. Fine coordinated movements are slightly reduced bilaterally. Gait consists of strides of normal length on a narrow base. Turning is more fluid and there is less tendency for freezing while turning. On pull test, he regains balance within one or two steps.

This case demonstrates a patient with motor fluctuations and dyskinesia. When OFF he has tremor and difficulty with ambulation, particularly turning. When ON, tremor resolves and gait is improved. However, his response is complicated by twisting, turning choreiform movements in the head and right hand.

Case 4. Post-traumatic Parkinsonism

This is a 53-year-old right-handed man with post-traumatic parkinsonism. Fifteen years ago, he was in an accident at work where two heavy metal doors swung down and caught his head in between. He suffered skull fractures on the right and facial fractures on the left. He was in the hospital for two weeks. When he recovered he had parkinsonism which slowly progressed over time, causing increased balance and gait difficulty. He has not responded to anti-parkinsonian medications. Videotaped examination reveals a moderate decrease in blink rate and facial expression. Voice is moderately soft. He has no rest, postural or kinetic tremors. Extra-ocular movements are normal. He has a right peripheral seventh nerve palsy causing right upper and lower facial weakness. He has decreased auditory perception on the right. Fine coordinated movements are moderately reduced bilaterally. He is able to arise from a chair with arms crossed with moderate slowness. Gait consists of strides of moderate to markedly shortened length. Turning is en bloc and requires many steps. Axial posture is mildly flexed. Arm swing during ambulation is absent bilaterally. On pull test, he takes many steps before regaining balance. This case demonstrates classic features of post-traumatic parkinsonism including absence of rest tremor and lack of response to dopamine medications.

Case 5. Subthalamic Nucleus (STN) Deep Brain Stimulation in a Patient with Parkinson's Disease

This is a 51-year-old man with a diagnosis of Parkinson's disease for eight years. He initially noticed tremor in the left arm and leg. He was treated with levodopa/carbidopa beginning eight years ago. He developed dyskinesias five years ago and wearing off motor fluctuations four years ago. He was OFF approximately 30% of the day and had dyskinesias 25% of the day. His was very disabled during OFF time and when dyskinetic. Because his motor fluctuations and dyskinesias could not be controlled with medications, he underwent bilateral subthalamic stimulation implants.

A. Examination in the OFF medication (medications withheld overnight) , OFF stimulator (stimulator turned off) state reveals a moderate decrease in blink rate and a marked decrease in facial expression. He has a moderate amplitude rest tremor in both hands and a mild tremor in the chin. With arms outstretched, he has a moderate postural tremor. He has mild slowness with finger tapping and hand movements bilaterally. He has moderate slowness on rapid alternating movements on both sides, left worse than right. Gait is slow with reduced strides with decrease in armswing bilaterally and tremor on the left side.

B. Examination while in the OFF medication, ON stimulator (stimulator turned on) state demonstrates resolution of tremor. Facial expression has improved. There is no slowness on finger tapping, hand movements or rapid alternating movements except for mild slowing on the left side. His gait is normal with good armswing bilaterally.

This case demonstrates a patient who has undergone bilateral subthalamic stimulation implants. When the devices are turned OFF he has tremor and difficulty with ambulation, particularly turning. When the devices are turned ON, tremor resolves and gait is improved.

Case 6. Thalamic Deep Brain Stimulation in a Patient with Essential Tremor

This is a 72-year-old woman with a history of essential tremor for 40 years. Her tremor progressively worsened over time and she developoed increased disability with activities of daily living. She underwent a left thalamic stimulator implant for improvement of right hand tremor. Videotaped examination with the thalamic stimulator turned off reveals the patient has a mild to moderate head tremor, mainly in the horizontal direction. She has severe postural tremor with the arms outstretched and kinetic tremor with movement, worse on the right side. She has severe tremor on finger-to-nose testing. She also has a mild rest tremor in the left upper extremity. Once the stimulator is turned on, she has marked improvement in the postural and kinetic tremor in her right hand along with some improvement in her head tremor. She can hold and pour from a cup with minimum difficulty and does not spill any water.

This case demonstrates a patient with essential tremor and shows how this condition is different from Parkinson's disease. She has undergone left brain thalamic stimulator implant. When the device is turned off, she has marked tremor and has difficulty with simple tasks such as pouring water. When the device is turned on, tremor is markedly reduced and she can pour water without spilling.

INDEX